Hope for Families

The Essential Caregiver's Guide to Supporting Loved Ones with POTS, MCAS, and EDS

Stella Marion Kaufman

Copyright © 2025 by Stella Marion Kaufman. All rights reserved.

First Edition: 2025

ISBN: 978-1-7642471-3-9

This book is intended for educational and informational purposes only. The content provided is not intended to replace professional medical advice, diagnosis, or treatment. Always seek the advice of your physician or other qualified healthcare providers with any questions you may have regarding a medical condition or treatment.

The author and publisher make no representations or warranties with respect to the accuracy or completeness of the contents of this work and specifically disclaim all warranties, including without limitation warranties of fitness for a particular purpose. The advice and strategies contained herein may not be suitable for every situation.

All names, characters, and case studies presented in this book are either fictitious or used with permission. Any resemblance to actual persons, living or deceased, or actual events is purely coincidental. Case examples are composites created for educational purposes and do not represent specific individuals or families.

References to medical professionals, healthcare institutions, and organizations are made for educational purposes only and do not constitute endorsements of this work or its contents.

The author disclaims any liability for any adverse effects arising from the use or application of the information contained in this book.

Table of Contents

Preface 1

Chapter 1: When Someone You Love Has Zebra Stripes 1
    Why These Conditions Are Called Invisible 1
    The Fluctuation Reality: Good Days and Bad Days 3
    Genetic Implications for Family Members 4
    Challenging Your Assumptions About Illness 4
    The Grief of Changing Relationships 5

Chapter 2: Medical Literacy for Families 8
    POTS, MCAS, and EDS Basics 8
    Common Symptoms and Presentations 9
    Treatment Approaches and Limitations 10
    Emergency Situations to Recognize 12
    Navigating Medical Appointments Together 12

Chapter 3: Daily Living Support 15
    Household Modifications and Safety 15
    Meal Planning for Dietary Restrictions 17
    Medication Management Assistance 19
    Transportation and Mobility Support 21
    Energy Conservation Partnership 22

Chapter 4: Emotional and Psychological Support 25
    Validation Without Fixing 25
    Listening Without Minimizing 27
    Managing Your Own Frustration 29
    Supporting Without Enabling 31
    Celebrating Small Victories 32

Chapter 5: Advocacy and Communication 35
Medical Advocacy Strategies 35
School and Workplace Support 37
Extended Family Education 39
Friend Group Dynamics 41
Public Situation Management 42

Chapter 6: Redefining Family Roles 45
When a Parent Is Ill 45
When a Child Is Ill 47
Sibling Dynamics and Support 49
Spouse and Partner Adjustments 51
Extended Family Involvement 52

Chapter 7: Financial and Practical Planning 55
Medical Expense Management 55
Insurance Navigation Together 57
Disability Application Support 59
Estate Planning Considerations 60
Emergency Planning 61

Chapter 8: Preventing Caregiver Burnout 64
Recognizing Burnout Signs 64
Setting Sustainable Boundaries 66
Building Support Networks 69
Respite Care Strategies 70
Maintaining Your Identity 72

Chapter 9: Relationship Preservation 75
Intimacy and Chronic Illness 75

Maintaining Friendship Within Caregiving 77
Date Nights and Connection 79
Managing Resentment 81
Growing Together Through Challenges 82
Chapter 10: Finding Meaning and Growth 85
Post-Traumatic Growth Possibilities 85
Building Family Resilience 87
Creating New Traditions 89
Advocacy and Community Involvement 91
Hope Without Toxic Positivity 93
References 96

Preface

A Letter to Families Walking This Path

The medical appointment that changed everything happened on a Tuesday. Your loved one walked into the doctor's office with symptoms that had puzzled physicians for months or years, and walked out with three diagnoses you'd never heard of: POTS, MCAS, and EDS. The relief of finally having answers quickly gave way to a flood of questions nobody seemed prepared to help you navigate.

You weren't the patient, but suddenly you became the researcher, the advocate, the crisis manager, and the emotional support system for conditions that most people—including many healthcare providers—don't understand. You found yourself drowning in medical terminology, insurance appeals, and the daily reality of supporting someone whose illness remains invisible to the outside world.

This book exists because families like yours have been overlooked in the chronic illness conversation for far too long.

Why This Book Matters

For decades, chronic illness resources have focused almost exclusively on patient experiences, leaving families to figure out their roles through trial and error. But here's what research consistently shows: family support dramatically impacts health outcomes for people with chronic conditions. When families understand these complex conditions and know how to provide effective support, everyone benefits—patients experience better symptom management, and families experience less stress and burnout.

Yet until now, no comprehensive guide existed specifically for families navigating POTS (Postural Orthostatic Tachycardia Syndrome), MCAS (Mast Cell Activation Syndrome), and EDS (Ehlers-Danlos Syndrome)—the trio of conditions often called "the trifecta" in chronic illness communities.

Your Family's Invisible Stripes

The title of this book, "Loving Someone with Invisible Stripes," reflects a profound truth about these conditions. Just as zebras earn their stripes through genetics, people with EDS carry invisible genetic variations that affect their connective tissue. These invisible stripes extend beyond the diagnosed individual to mark entire families who must adapt, advocate, and learn to thrive despite chronic illness challenges.

Your family now carries invisible stripes too—the marks of resilience, adaptation, and love that develop when chronic illness becomes part of your story. These stripes aren't scars; they're evidence of your commitment to supporting someone you love through circumstances you never expected to face.

What Makes This Guide Different

This book approaches chronic illness from your perspective—the family member who didn't choose this journey but finds yourself walking it anyway. Every chapter acknowledges that you have your own needs, limitations, and emotions that deserve attention and support.

You'll find practical guidance that goes beyond basic medical information to address real-world challenges: What do you do when your child's teacher doesn't believe their symptoms are real? How do you manage family finances when medical expenses spiral beyond your budget? How do you maintain your marriage when chronic illness affects intimacy and shared activities? How do you prevent caregiver burnout while providing the support your loved one needs?

Built on Real Experience

The strategies, case examples, and guidance in this book come from extensive research combined with real stories from families who have navigated these exact challenges. Every recommendation has been tested in the complex reality of daily life with chronic illness, not just theoretical medical settings.

The families whose experiences inform this work have generously shared their struggles, mistakes, breakthroughs, and hard-won wisdom so that your family doesn't have to navigate this path alone. Their stories become your roadmap for building effective support systems while maintaining your own well-being.

A Community of Understanding

Reading this book connects you to a larger community of families who understand the unique challenges of supporting someone with invisible chronic illness. You'll discover that the feelings you've experienced—the fear, frustration, grief, and eventual acceptance—are normal parts of the family adjustment process.

More importantly, you'll learn that families can not only survive chronic illness but find meaning, growth, and deeper connections through the process of adapting together. The journey isn't easy, but it's not hopeless. With the right knowledge, tools, and support, your family can build a life that accommodates chronic illness while still pursuing joy, purpose, and connection.

How to Use This Guide

This book is designed to meet you wherever you are in your family's chronic illness journey. If you're newly diagnosed and feeling overwhelmed, start with Chapters 1 and 2 to build foundational understanding. If you're struggling with daily management, focus on Chapters 3 through 5 for practical strategies. If you're experiencing relationship stress or caregiver burnout, Chapters 8 and 9 provide essential support.

Feel free to read chapters out of order based on your family's immediate needs. Each chapter stands alone while contributing to a larger framework for successful family adaptation to chronic illness.

An Invitation to Hope

This preface comes with an invitation—not to false optimism that ignores real challenges, but to evidence-based hope grounded in the experiences of families who have walked this path before you. They've discovered that love, armed with knowledge and practical skills, can create support systems that transform chronic illness from a family crisis into a manageable part of a meaningful life.

Your family's story with invisible stripes is just beginning. This book provides the guidance, tools, and encouragement you need to write that story with confidence, compassion, and hope for the future.

You're not alone in this journey. Your love matters. Your support makes a difference. And your family has the strength to not just survive these challenges, but to thrive despite them.

With understanding and hope for your family's path ahead,

Stella Marion Kaufman

If this book helps your family in any way, please consider sharing your experience with other families who might benefit from these resources. Together, we can ensure that no family has to navigate invisible chronic illness without support, understanding, and practical guidance.

Chapter 1: When Someone You Love Has Zebra Stripes

The diagnosis letter sits on the kitchen table, medical terms swimming across the page like a foreign language. Your loved one has just been told they have POTS, MCAS, and EDS—conditions you've never heard of before today. The doctor mentioned something about "zebras," and you're wondering what wild animals have to do with your family member's mysterious symptoms that have puzzled physicians for years.

This moment marks the beginning of a journey that will reshape how you understand illness, health, and the very nature of being sick in America. Unlike the clear-cut broken bones or obvious infections you've encountered before, these conditions operate in shadows, fluctuating like tides, appearing and disappearing without warning (Bryarly et al., 2019).

Why These Conditions Are Called Invisible

The medical community borrowed a phrase from diagnostic training: "When you hear hoofbeats, think horses, not zebras." This saying teaches doctors to consider common conditions first—the horses of medicine. But for patients with POTS (Postural Orthostatic Tachycardia Syndrome), MCAS (Mast Cell Activation Syndrome), and EDS (Ehlers-Danlos Syndrome), they are the zebras—rare, complex, and often misunderstood (Kohn et al., 2021).

These conditions earn the "invisible" label because their symptoms don't show up in typical ways. Your loved one might look perfectly healthy while experiencing heart rates that soar to 140 beats per minute just from standing up. They might smile during a family dinner while their body launches an internal allergic reaction to the very air they're breathing. The absence of obvious external signs creates a unique challenge for families trying to understand what's really happening.

Case Example 1: Sarah's Story

Sarah, a 28-year-old teacher, spent three years visiting different specialists before receiving her trifecta diagnosis. Her family watched her transform from an active, energetic person to someone who needed help carrying groceries. Her mother, Janet, recalls the frustration: "She looked fine to everyone else. People would say, 'But you don't look sick,' and I could see how much that hurt her. I started questioning if maybe she was just stressed or depressed."

The invisibility factor created tension within Sarah's family. Her younger brother assumed she was "making excuses" to avoid family gatherings, while her father wondered if she needed psychiatric help rather than medical treatment. Only after attending medical appointments with Sarah did Janet begin to understand that her daughter's body was fighting battles no one could see.

Case Example 2: Marcus and His Teenage Son

Fifteen-year-old David began experiencing severe fatigue and joint pain during his sophomore year of high school. His father, Marcus, initially attributed the symptoms to typical teenage behavior. "I thought he was just being lazy or trying to get out of chores," Marcus admits. "When he'd say he was too tired to walk the dog, I'd get frustrated and tell him to toughen up."

The turning point came when David collapsed during a basketball game. Emergency room tests revealed a heart rate of 160 after standing for just two minutes. The cardiologist's explanation of POTS opened Marcus's eyes to the fact that his son's complaints weren't behavioral issues but legitimate medical symptoms that had been hiding in plain sight.

Research shows that patients with invisible chronic illnesses face unique psychosocial challenges, including disbelief from family members and social isolation (Åsbring & Närvänen, 2020). The lack of visible symptoms creates what researchers call "diagnostic limbo"—a period where families struggle to understand and validate experiences that don't match their expectations of illness.

The Fluctuation Reality: Good Days and Bad Days

Traditional concepts of illness follow predictable patterns: you get sick, you get treatment, you recover. Chronic conditions with invisible symptoms operate by entirely different rules. Your loved one might wake up feeling relatively normal, enjoy lunch with friends, then spend the evening unable to stand without assistance. This unpredictability creates confusion for families accustomed to linear health experiences.

The fluctuating nature of these conditions means planning becomes nearly impossible. Family events get cancelled at the last minute. Work schedules require constant adjustments. Social commitments become sources of anxiety rather than joy. Understanding this reality requires a fundamental shift in how you think about health and illness (Kohn et al., 2021).

Case Example 3: The Williams Family Vacation

The Williams family planned a week-long beach vacation for two years. Lisa, their 24-year-old daughter with the trifecta, felt optimistic about the trip during her "good phase" in spring. However, two days before departure, a MCAS flare triggered by seasonal allergens left her unable to travel. The family faced a difficult choice: cancel the entire vacation or leave Lisa behind.

"We decided to stay home," explains her mother, Carol. "But I could see the guilt in Lisa's eyes. She felt responsible for ruining everyone's plans. That's when we realized we needed to approach family activities differently. We started planning backup options and shorter trips that could be modified based on how she was feeling."

This experience taught the Williams family that flexibility isn't just helpful—it's essential. They learned to celebrate good days without taking them for granted and support bad days without resentment.

The fluctuating nature of symptoms creates what medical professionals call "the uncertainty principle" in chronic illness management (Marton et al., 2021). Families must learn to live with ambiguity while maintaining hope and planning for the future.

Genetic Implications for Family Members

EDS is a hereditary condition, which means other family members may carry the same genetic variations. This discovery often triggers a cascade of realizations as relatives begin connecting their own unexplained symptoms to a larger genetic picture. The aunt who always had "loose joints," the grandfather with recurring digestive issues, or the cousin with frequent headaches might all share the same underlying condition.

Learning about genetic implications creates both relief and anxiety within families. Relief comes from finally having explanations for seemingly unrelated health issues that have puzzled family members for years. Anxiety emerges from concerns about children and grandchildren who might inherit these conditions (Castori et al., 2019).

The genetic component also means families must make decisions about testing other members. Some relatives want immediate answers, while others prefer not to know. These conversations require sensitivity and understanding that each person's approach to genetic information differs.

Parents of children with EDS often experience guilt, wondering if they "passed on" the condition. Adult children worry about having biological children of their own. Extended families sometimes struggle with blame or misunderstanding about genetic inheritance patterns.

Challenging Your Assumptions About Illness

Most families operate with unspoken assumptions about health and sickness. We expect sick people to stay in bed, to get better with rest, to follow predictable recovery patterns. These conditions challenge every assumption you've held about illness and recovery.

Your loved one might need to lie down after a shower but feel energetic enough to work on a creative project later the same day. They might require a wheelchair for grocery shopping but manage to walk normally at home. These apparent contradictions aren't signs of inconsistency or exaggeration—they reflect the complex nature of conditions that affect multiple body systems simultaneously.

Family members often struggle with the concept that someone can be simultaneously sick and functional, disabled and capable, struggling and successful. This cognitive dissonance requires time and education to resolve (Bryarly et al., 2019).

Understanding these conditions requires accepting that traditional cause-and-effect relationships don't apply. Rest doesn't always bring improvement. Exercise doesn't always increase strength. Positive thinking doesn't overcome physiological limitations. This acceptance challenges deeply held cultural beliefs about health, recovery, and personal responsibility.

The Grief of Changing Relationships

Chronic illness affects entire family systems, not just the diagnosed individual. The person you knew—your energetic daughter, your adventurous spouse, your active parent—may seem fundamentally changed by their condition. This change triggers a grief process that many families don't expect or understand.

You might grieve the loss of shared activities that are no longer possible. Family hiking trips, shopping marathons, or spontaneous adventures may become memories rather than ongoing traditions. The grief extends to future plans and dreams that now require modification or abandonment.

This grief is complicated because your loved one is still present, still the same person, but their capacity and energy have changed. The person remains while the relationship dynamics shift, creating a unique form of loss that isn't recognized in traditional grief models (Marton et al., 2021).

Family members often experience guilt about grieving these changes, feeling selfish for focusing on their own losses when their loved one is the one facing daily symptoms. This guilt compounds the grief and can lead to emotional isolation within the family system.

The grief process includes anger—at the medical system that took years to provide answers, at the unpredictability of symptoms, at the limitations now imposed on family life. Bargaining appears in the form of searching for miracle cures or perfect treatments. Depression emerges as the reality of chronic, incurable conditions settles in.

Acceptance doesn't mean giving up hope for improvement or adaptation. Instead, it means integrating the reality of these conditions into your family's new normal while maintaining love, support, and connection through the challenges.

Reflections on Understanding

The journey of understanding invisible chronic illness requires patience, education, and a willingness to challenge long-held beliefs about health and sickness. Your loved one with zebra stripes isn't broken or defective—they're managing complex medical conditions that require different approaches to daily living and family dynamics.

Recognition that these conditions are real, unpredictable, and life-altering forms the foundation for building effective support systems. The invisibility of symptoms doesn't diminish their impact or validity. The fluctuating nature of good and bad days requires flexibility and understanding rather than frustration or disbelief.

Moving beyond traditional concepts of illness toward acceptance of chronic, invisible conditions opens the door to deeper compassion and more effective family support. Your loved one needs allies who understand that their zebra stripes are part of their reality, not a choice or a phase to overcome.

Key Insights to Remember:

- Invisible conditions are medically complex, not imaginary or psychological
- Symptom fluctuation is characteristic of these conditions, not inconsistency
- Genetic components affect entire families, not just diagnosed individuals
- Grief over relationship changes is normal and expected
- Understanding requires challenging assumptions about illness and recovery
- Support begins with believing and validating your loved one's experiences

Chapter 2: Medical Literacy for Families

Standing in the cardiologist's office, you listen as medical terms flow like water from a broken dam: "orthostatic intolerance," "tachycardia," "small fiber neuropathy," "mast cell degranulation." The doctor speaks quickly, assumingfamiliarity with concepts that sound like a foreign language. Your loved one nods along, but you see the same confusion in their eyes that you feel in your chest.

Medical literacy becomes a survival skill when chronic, complex conditions enter your family. You need more than basic understanding—you need working knowledge that helps you advocate, support, and navigate a healthcare system that often struggles with these conditions itself (Kohn et al., 2021).

POTS, MCAS, and EDS Basics

POTS affects the autonomic nervous system—the network that controls automatic body functions like heart rate, blood pressure, and temperature regulation. Think of it as your body's internal thermostat and circulation system malfunctioning. When a person with POTS stands up, their heart rate increases excessively (typically 30 beats per minute or more) to compensate for blood pooling in their legs (Bryarly et al., 2019).

The autonomic nervous system normally adjusts blood flow seamlessly as you move from lying down to standing. In POTS, this adjustment fails, creating symptoms like dizziness, rapid heartbeat, fatigue, and brain fog. These symptoms aren't character flaws or anxiety responses—they're physiological reactions to a malfunctioning autonomic system.

MCAS involves mast cells—immune system cells that release chemicals like histamine during allergic reactions. In MCAS, these cells become hyperactive, releasing chemicals inappropriately and causing symptoms throughout the body. Unlike typical allergies with

8

obvious triggers, MCAS can cause reactions to heat, cold, stress, foods, chemicals, or seemingly nothing at all (Weinstock et al., 2021).

Mast cells exist in every organ system, which explains why MCAS symptoms can affect digestion, breathing, skin, cardiovascular function, and neurological processes simultaneously. Your loved one isn't having multiple unrelated problems—they're experiencing one condition that affects multiple systems.

EDS affects connective tissue—the "glue" that holds body structures together. Collagen, a protein that provides strength and flexibility to skin, joints, blood vessels, and organs, doesn't form properly in EDS. This creates joint hypermobility, skin changes, and problems with internal organs that depend on strong connective tissue (Castori et al., 2019).

Case Example 1: Understanding Maria's Daily Reality

Maria's family struggled to understand why she needed to sit down frequently during shopping trips until they learned about blood pooling in POTS. Her mother, Carmen, describes the revelation: "The doctor explained that Maria's blood doesn't circulate properly when she stands. It pools in her legs, so her heart has to work overtime just to get blood to her brain. No wonder she gets exhausted from simple activities that don't bother the rest of us."

Understanding the physiology behind Maria's symptoms changed how her family approached daily activities. Instead of interpreting her need to sit as weakness or laziness, they recognized it as a medical necessity and began planning activities around her body's actual limitations.

Common Symptoms and Presentations

These conditions rarely present in isolation. Most patients experience overlapping symptoms that create complex clinical pictures. Understanding common presentations helps families recognize patterns and communicate effectively with healthcare providers.

POTS symptoms typically worsen with standing, heat, exercise, stress, and hormonal changes. Common presentations include rapid heartbeat upon standing, dizziness, fatigue that's disproportionate to activity level, brain fog, nausea, and exercise intolerance. Sleep disturbances are common, as is difficulty regulating body temperature (Bryarly et al., 2019).

MCAS symptoms can affect any organ system and may include flushing, hives, digestive issues, breathing difficulties, fatigue, brain fog, anxiety-like symptoms, and severe reactions to foods, chemicals, or environmental triggers. The unpredictable nature of MCAS reactions creates significant lifestyle challenges (Weinstock et al., 2021).

EDS symptoms include joint hypermobility, frequent dislocations or subluxations, easy bruising, skin that's soft or stretchy, slow wound healing, digestive problems, and chronic pain. Many patients also experience fatigue and sleep disturbances related to pain and joint instability (Castori et al., 2019).

Case Example 2: Recognizing Patterns in Jake's Symptoms

Jake's parents spent months taking him to different specialists—dermatology for his skin issues, gastroenterology for digestive problems, orthopedics for joint pain. His father, Robert, recalls the confusion: "Each doctor focused on their specialty, but no one was looking at the bigger picture. Jake's skin problems, stomach issues, and joint pain all seemed unrelated until we found a doctor who understood connective tissue disorders."

The pattern recognition came when Jake's mother started keeping a detailed symptom diary. She noticed that his worst days included multiple symptoms across different body systems, suggesting a common underlying cause rather than separate conditions.

Treatment Approaches and Limitations

Treatment for these conditions focuses on symptom management rather than cures. This reality requires families to adjust expectations and understand that improvement is measured in quality of life rather than complete recovery.

POTS treatment typically includes increasing fluid and salt intake, compression garments, medications to support blood pressure and heart rate, and carefully planned exercise programs. The goal is managing symptoms to improve function rather than eliminating the condition (Kohn et al., 2021).

MCAS treatment involves identifying and avoiding triggers when possible, medications to stabilize mast cells and block their chemical releases, and emergency medications for severe reactions. Treatment is highly individualized because triggers and responses vary significantly between patients (Weinstock et al., 2021).

EDS treatment focuses on protecting joints, managing pain, and preventing complications. Physical therapy, bracing, pain management, and careful monitoring of cardiovascular and digestive complications form the treatment foundation. Surgery is sometimes necessary but carries additional risks due to connective tissue fragility (Castori et al., 2019).

Case Example 3: Managing Treatment Expectations

The Henderson family initially expected quick results from treatment, assuming that proper medication would "fix" their daughter Emma's POTS. Her mother, Linda, explains their learning process: "We thought the doctor would prescribe something and Emma would go back to normal. It took months to understand that treatment is about finding the right combination of medications, lifestyle changes, and accommodations that help her function better, not about curing the condition."

This realization helped the family develop realistic expectations and celebrate small improvements rather than waiting for dramatic changes. They learned to measure success in terms of Emma's ability to participate in activities she enjoyed rather than comparing her to healthy peers.

Emergency Situations to Recognize

Understanding when symptoms require immediate medical attention protects your loved one and prevents unnecessary emergency room visits for manageable symptoms. However, these conditions can create genuine emergencies that require prompt recognition and response.

POTS emergencies might include severe dehydration, fainting with injury, chest pain, or symptoms that don't respond to usual management strategies. High fever can worsen POTS symptoms significantly and may require medical intervention (Bryarly et al., 2019).

MCAS can cause anaphylaxis—a severe, life-threatening allergic reaction that requires immediate emergency treatment. Warning signs include difficulty breathing, swelling of face or throat, severe full-body hives, vomiting, diarrhea, and loss of consciousness. Patients at risk for anaphylaxis typically carry epinephrine auto-injectors (Weinstock et al., 2021).

EDS emergencies might include organ rupture (particularly hollow organs like intestines or blood vessels), pneumothorax (collapsed lung), or severe injuries from joint dislocations. The fragile connective tissue in EDS can create complications that wouldn't occur in people with normal collagen structure (Castori et al., 2019).

Families need written emergency action plans that outline specific symptoms requiring immediate medical attention, medications to administer, and information to provide to emergency responders who may be unfamiliar with these conditions.

Navigating Medical Appointments Together

Medical appointments become more productive when family members understand how to prepare, participate, and follow up effectively. Your role extends beyond transportation to active advocacy and support.

Preparation involves organizing symptoms, questions, and medical history before appointments. Many specialists have limited time and may not be familiar with the complexity of these conditions. Bringing organized information helps maximize appointment effectiveness.

During appointments, family members can help by taking notes, asking clarifying questions, and advocating for thorough evaluation. Many patients experience brain fog or feel overwhelmed during medical visits, making a supportive family member valuable for information retention and communication.

Following up after appointments ensures that treatment plans are implemented correctly and that concerning symptoms receive appropriate attention. Many treatment adjustments require ongoing communication with healthcare providers rather than waiting for the next scheduled appointment.

Building relationships with healthcare providers who understand these conditions creates a foundation for long-term management. These relationships often require time and persistence but provide essential support for complex medical needs.

Clinical Perspectives on Family Involvement

The most successful treatment outcomes occur when families develop medical literacy that supports their loved one without overwhelming them. Understanding the basics of these conditions helps families provide appropriate support, recognize concerning symptoms, and advocate effectively within the healthcare system.

Medical literacy isn't about becoming medical experts—it's about understanding enough to be effective advocates and supportive family members. This knowledge empowers families to ask appropriate questions, recognize treatment progress or setbacks, and participate meaningfully in medical decision-making.

The complexity of these conditions requires ongoing learning and adaptation. Medical understanding develops over time through experience, education, and communication with healthcare providers who specialize in these areas.

Essential Knowledge for Moving Ahead:

- These conditions affect multiple body systems simultaneously, not separately
- Treatment focuses on symptom management and quality of life improvement
- Emergency situations require specific recognition and response protocols
- Medical appointments benefit from preparation, participation, and follow-up
- Ongoing medical literacy supports long-term management and advocacy
- Understanding physiology behind symptoms reduces family confusion and increases support

Chapter 3: Daily Living Support

The morning routine that once took twenty minutes now stretches to an hour and a half. Your loved one sits on the shower bench, heart rate climbing as hot water streams down, while you gather compression stockings and prepare a saltwater drink for after they towel off. The simple act of getting ready for the day has become a carefully orchestrated dance between symptoms and solutions.

Daily living with POTS, MCAS, and EDS requires fundamental changes to how households operate. The modifications aren't just helpful suggestions—they become necessary accommodations that determine your loved one's ability to function safely and comfortably at home. These adaptations extend beyond the physical environment to include meal planning, medication schedules, transportation arrangements, and energy management strategies that affect every family member (Bryarly et al., 2019).

Household Modifications and Safety

Home safety takes on new dimensions when connective tissue disorders and dysautonomia enter the picture. Traditional home hazards become amplified risks, while new safety concerns emerge that most families never consider.

Bathroom Safety Modifications

The bathroom poses particular challenges for people with these conditions. Hot showers can trigger POTS symptoms by causing blood vessel dilation and blood pooling. Installing a shower chair or bench allows your loved one to sit during showers, reducing the risk of fainting and falls. Temperature regulation becomes critical—lukewarm water prevents symptom flares while still providing adequate cleaning.

Grab bars positioned strategically near the toilet, shower, and bathtub provide stability for someone with EDS whose joints may give way unexpectedly. These aren't just for elderly people—young adults with hypermobile joints need reliable support points to prevent injury during routine activities.

Non-slip mats and textured surfaces reduce fall risks for people who experience dizziness or joint instability. The investment in bathroom safety modifications pays dividends in preventing emergency room visits and maintaining independence in personal care activities.

Kitchen Adaptations for Safety and Function

Kitchen modifications focus on reducing the physical demands of meal preparation while maintaining safety. Lower shelves store frequently used items to minimize reaching overhead, which can trigger POTS symptoms. Lightweight cookware reduces joint stress for people with EDS, while ergonomic handles accommodate hypermobile fingers and wrists.

Installing pullout drawers and lazy Susans eliminates the need to bend deeply or reach into dark corners where joint positioning becomes awkward and potentially harmful. Good lighting prevents eye strain and reduces the risk of accidents during food preparation.

Counter-height seating allows cooking while sitting, conserving energy and reducing orthostatic stress. Many people with POTS find that standing for extended periods while cooking triggers symptoms, making seated food preparation a practical necessity rather than a luxury.

Case Example 1: The Martinez Family Kitchen Revolution

Elena Martinez was diagnosed with the trifecta at age 32, just as she and her husband were renovating their kitchen. Initially, they planned a typical remodel with high cabinets and standard appliances. Elena's mother, Rosa, pushed for modifications that seemed unnecessary at the time.

"I thought Mom was being overly cautious," recalls Elena's husband, Carlos. "Elena looked fine, and we didn't understand how much her conditions would affect daily activities. Six months later, Elena could barely stand long enough to make coffee, let alone prepare family meals."

The family retrofitted their new kitchen with pull-down shelving, a kitchen island with seating, and reorganized storage to keep essential items within easy reach. They added a small refrigerator at counter height to eliminate bending for frequently used items. These modifications transformed meal preparation from an exhausting ordeal into a manageable activity.

Rosa's foresight proved valuable when Elena's symptoms worsened during a medication adjustment period. The kitchen adaptations allowed her to maintain some independence in meal preparation even during her most symptomatic phases.

Meal Planning for Dietary Restrictions

MCAS creates complex dietary challenges that extend far beyond typical food allergies. Triggers can include natural food chemicals, additives, preservatives, and even cooking methods. Meal planning becomes a careful balance between nutrition, safety, and practicality for the entire family.

Understanding MCAS Dietary Restrictions

MCAS dietary restrictions often include histamine-rich foods, which encompass many common ingredients like aged cheeses, fermented foods, citrus fruits, tomatoes, and leftover meats. These restrictions eliminate entire food categories that form the foundation of typical family meals.

Food preparation methods also matter in MCAS management. Fresh foods are generally safer than leftovers, which accumulate histamine during storage. This reality means meal planning must account for immediate consumption rather than preparing large batches for the week.

Cross-contamination becomes a serious concern in MCAS households. Even trace amounts of trigger foods can cause reactions, requiring separate preparation areas, utensils, and storage containers for safe foods.

Practical Meal Planning Strategies

Successful meal planning for MCAS starts with identifying safe foods through systematic elimination diets guided by knowledgeable healthcare providers. Building a core list of tolerated foods provides the foundation for meal rotation and family menu planning.

Batch cooking safe foods during good symptom days creates reserves for difficult periods. Freezing individual portions of tolerated meals provides quick options during flares when cooking becomes challenging or impossible.

Family meal coordination requires creativity and flexibility. Many families find success in preparing base ingredients that can be customized for different dietary needs. For example, plain grilled chicken can be seasoned differently for family members with and without MCAS restrictions.

Case Example 2: The Thompson Family Mealtime Transformation

When 16-year-old Michael Thompson developed severe MCAS reactions to most family foods, his mother Sarah felt overwhelmed by the dietary restrictions. Michael's safe food list included fewer than twenty items, none of which appealed to his younger siblings.

"I was cooking three different meals every night," Sarah explains. "Michael needed fresh, low-histamine foods. His little sister wanted normal kid foods. My husband worked long hours and needed quick, filling meals. I felt like a short-order cook in my own kitchen."

The family worked with a nutritionist familiar with MCAS to develop a rotation meal plan that accommodated everyone's needs. They identified base proteins and vegetables that Michael could tolerate, then created family meals around these foundations. Spices and sauces were added individually to accommodate different preferences and restrictions.

The solution involved more planning but less actual cooking time. Sarah prepared larger quantities of Michael's safe foods and froze portions for quick reheating. The family discovered new foods they enjoyed while supporting Michael's dietary needs.

Medication Management Assistance

Complex medication regimens become the norm for people managing POTS, MCAS, and EDS. Multiple prescriptions, supplements, timing requirements, and dosage adjustments create management challenges that benefit from family support and organization systems.

Organizing Complex Medication Schedules

Many people with these conditions take medications multiple times daily, with specific timing requirements related to meals, activities, or other medications. Creating visual medication schedules helps ensure nothing gets missed during brain fog episodes or particularly symptomatic days.

Pill organizers become essential tools, but the standard weekly organizers often prove inadequate for complex regimens. Multiple daily doses, liquid medications, and refrigerated items require sophisticated organization systems that accommodate the reality of polypharmacy.

Backup systems prove crucial during emergencies or travel. Maintaining current medication lists, dosage information, and prescribing physician contacts ensures continuity of care during medical emergencies or when seeing unfamiliar healthcare providers.

Supporting Medication Adherence

Family members can assist with medication management without taking complete control. This balance maintains the patient's autonomy while providing necessary support during difficult periods.

Medication reminders help during brain fog episodes or particularly symptomatic days when cognitive function becomes impaired. These reminders can range from simple verbal prompts to sophisticated smartphone apps that track timing and adherence.

Pharmacy coordination becomes complex when multiple specialists prescribe different medications. Family members can help track prescriptions, manage refills, and communicate with pharmacies about timing and insurance issues.

Case Example 3: Managing Rebecca's Medication Regiment

Rebecca Chen's medication schedule included twelve different prescriptions and supplements taken at various times throughout the day. Her husband, David, initially tried to manage everything for her, creating tension and reducing Rebecca's sense of control over her own care.

"David meant well, but I felt like a child being managed rather than an adult managing a medical condition," Rebecca explains. "We had to find a balance between his help and my independence."

The couple developed a collaborative system where Rebecca maintained primary responsibility for her medications while David provided backup support. They used a combination of smartphone apps, weekly pill organizers, and shared calendars to track doses and timing.

David's role evolved to include pharmacy runs, insurance coordination, and emergency backup during Rebecca's worst symptom days. This division of responsibilities supported Rebecca's independence while ensuring her complex medication needs were met consistently.

Transportation and Mobility Support

Transportation challenges affect not just the person with these conditions but entire family schedules and logistics. Driving limitations, public transportation difficulties, and mobility needs require creative solutions and family coordination.

Driving Limitations and Alternatives

POTS can affect driving safety through symptoms like dizziness, brain fog, and fatigue. Many people with these conditions experience periods when driving becomes unsafe, requiring alternative transportation arrangements.

Family members often become primary drivers by default, but this arrangement can create resentment and logistical challenges. Planning transportation needs in advance helps prevent last-minute scrambling and reduces stress for everyone involved.

Ride-sharing services provide independence for people who can't drive during symptomatic periods. However, the cost of frequent ride-sharing can strain family budgets, making public transportation or family coordination more practical long-term solutions.

Mobility Aids and Equipment

Mobility aids often become necessary during symptom flares or for specific activities. Wheelchairs, walking aids, and compression garments help maintain function and independence during challenging periods.

The decision to use mobility aids can be emotionally difficult for both patients and families. Young adults particularly struggle with the visible acknowledgment of disability that mobility aids represent. Family support during these transitions proves crucial for acceptance and appropriate use.

Mobility equipment requires storage, maintenance, and transportation considerations that affect the entire family. Cars may need modifications to accommodate wheelchairs or walking aids. Home storage space must be allocated for equipment that may only be used periodically.

Energy Conservation Partnership

Energy management becomes a family affair when chronic illness affects daily functioning. Understanding energy conservation principles helps families support their loved one while maintaining household routines and responsibilities.

Understanding Energy Limitations

The energy limitations experienced in these conditions differ from normal fatigue. This isn't tiredness that improves with rest—it's a fundamental limitation in the body's ability to produce and sustain energy for normal activities (Bryarly et al., 2019).

Spoon theory provides a useful framework for understanding energy limitations. Each person starts the day with a limited number of "spoons" representing energy units. Activities consume spoons, and once they're gone, rest is required before more energy becomes available.

Family members benefit from understanding that energy conservation isn't laziness or lack of motivation. It's a medical necessity that prevents symptom flares and maintains function over the long term.

Family Energy Management Strategies

Redistributing household responsibilities allows the family member with chronic illness to conserve energy for essential activities. This redistribution requires honest communication about capabilities and limitations without judgment or resentment.

Flexible scheduling accommodates the unpredictable nature of energy levels in these conditions. Family plans must include backup options for when energy levels don't support originally planned activities.

Celebrating energy-efficient accomplishments helps maintain morale while acknowledging the reality of energy limitations. Success gets measured differently when chronic illness affects the family—completing a single task well may represent a significant achievement.

Practical Implementation Wisdom

The most successful families approach daily living support as a collaborative effort rather than a caregiver-patient relationship. This collaboration maintains dignity and independence while providing necessary assistance during challenging periods.

Flexibility remains the key to successful adaptation. What works during stable periods may need modification during symptom flares or medication adjustments. Families that remain adaptable find better long-term success than those who rigidly adhere to single solutions.

Communication about needs, limitations, and frustrations prevents resentment from building within family systems. Regular family meetings about practical needs and emotional challenges help maintain healthy relationships while managing chronic illness demands.

Essential Practical Knowledge

- Home modifications prevent injuries and enable independence for people with these conditions
- Meal planning for MCAS requires understanding histamine reactions and cross-contamination prevention
- Medication management benefits from family support while maintaining patient autonomy
- Transportation needs require planning and flexibility to accommodate driving limitations
- Energy conservation principles guide daily activity planning and family responsibility distribution

- Successful adaptations require ongoing communication and willingness to modify approaches as conditions change

Chapter 4: Emotional and Psychological Support

The text message arrives at 2 AM: "Having a bad day. Feel like I'm failing everyone." Your loved one with invisible chronic illness sits in their bedroom, overwhelmed by symptoms you can't see and emotions they struggle to express. The impulse to fix, to offer solutions, to minimize their distress feels overwhelming—but these well-meaning responses often create more isolation than support.

Emotional support for someone with POTS, MCAS, and EDS requires skills that feel counterintuitive to most family members. The natural desire to help by solving problems can inadvertently invalidate experiences and create emotional distance precisely when connection becomes most crucial (Marton et al., 2021).

Validation Without Fixing

Validation means acknowledging and accepting someone's emotional experience without immediately trying to change or solve it. For families dealing with chronic invisible illness, this skill becomes foundational to maintaining emotional connection and trust.

The Difference Between Validation and Agreement

Validating someone's emotions doesn't mean agreeing with their conclusions or perspectives. You can acknowledge that your loved one feels overwhelmed without agreeing that they're actually failing at everything. You can recognize their frustration without accepting that their situation is hopeless.

This distinction allows family members to provide emotional support while maintaining their own perspective. You're not required to adopt your loved one's emotional state or worldview to offer meaningful validation.

Validation focuses on the feeling rather than the content. Instead of debating facts or offering alternative perspectives, validation acknowledges the emotional reality your loved one is experiencing in the moment.

Practical Validation Techniques

Reflective listening forms the foundation of validation. This involves repeating back what you hear your loved one saying, both factually and emotionally. "It sounds like you're feeling frustrated because your symptoms made it impossible to finish your project today."

Normalizing responses help your loved one understand that their emotional reactions make sense given their circumstances. "Of course you feel disappointed—you were looking forward to that event for weeks, and missing it because of a flare is genuinely disappointing."

Avoiding the urge to immediately offer perspective or solutions allows your loved one to feel heard before moving toward problem-solving. Many situations benefit from validation first, solutions later—sometimes much later.

Case Example 1: Learning to Validate Jessica's Experience

Jessica's father, Mark, struggled with validation after her POTS diagnosis. His natural problem-solving approach led him to offer suggestions every time Jessica expressed frustration about her symptoms or limitations.

"Dad would immediately start listing things I could try—different doctors, new medications, lifestyle changes," Jessica recalls. "He meant well, but it made me feel like he thought I wasn't trying hard enough or that my problems were simple to fix."

The turning point came during a family therapy session where Mark learned the difference between validation and problem-solving. He practiced simply acknowledging Jessica's difficult experiences without immediately jumping to solutions.

"Learning to say 'That sounds really hard' instead of 'Have you tried...' was harder than I expected," Mark admits. "But I noticed Jessica started talking to me more when she felt heard rather than managed."

This shift improved their relationship significantly. Jessica felt more supported, and Mark felt more helpful even though he was doing less active problem-solving.

Listening Without Minimizing

Minimizing happens when family members unconsciously reduce the significance of their loved one's experiences through comparison, perspective-giving, or positive reframing attempts. These responses, while well-intended, can create emotional distance and reduce trust in family relationships.

Common Minimizing Patterns

Comparison minimizing occurs when family members point out others who have worse situations. "At least you don't have cancer" or "Think about people who are paralyzed" might be factually accurate but emotionally invalidating for someone struggling with daily symptoms.

Perspective minimizing happens when family members offer unsolicited positive reframes. "Look on the bright side—at least you have a diagnosis now" might be meant to encourage but can make your loved one feel misunderstood or judged for not being more positive.

Temporal minimizing involves suggesting that current difficulties are temporary or not significant in the long term. "This too shall pass" or "You'll feel better tomorrow" may dismiss the present reality of suffering.

The Impact of Minimizing on Relationships

Chronic minimizing teaches your loved one that their experiences aren't acceptable to share with family members. Over time, this leads to emotional withdrawal and increased isolation during difficult periods.

People learn to filter their communications when they expect minimizing responses. They may stop sharing struggles entirely or only present sanitized versions of their experiences that don't trigger family discomfort.

The person offering minimizing often feels frustrated because their attempts to help seem ineffective or unwelcome. This creates a negative cycle where both parties feel misunderstood and disconnected.

Alternatives to Minimizing Responses

Acknowledging the difficulty of your loved one's situation without immediately trying to improve their perspective creates space for authentic emotional expression. "This situation really is challenging" validates their experience.

Asking questions about their experience demonstrates genuine interest in understanding rather than changing their perspective. "What's the hardest part about dealing with this flare?" shows you want to understand their specific struggles.

Sitting with discomfort allows your loved one to process difficult emotions without feeling pressure to feel better quickly. Sometimes the most supportive response is simply "I'm here with you in this."

Case Example 2: The Garcia Family's Communication Transformation

When 19-year-old Sofia Garcia was diagnosed with EDS and MCAS, her mother Carmen's initial response involved constant positive reframing. Carmen couldn't tolerate seeing Sofia struggle and consistently offered optimistic perspectives on every difficulty.

"Mom would say things like 'At least we know what's wrong now' or 'Many people manage these conditions well,'" Sofia explains. "I felt like I couldn't be upset or scared without disappointing her."

Carmen's minimizing came from love and anxiety about Sofia's future. She believed that maintaining positivity would help Sofia cope better with her conditions. However, Sofia began withdrawing from family conversations and spending more time alone.

A family counselor helped Carmen understand that Sofia needed space to process the grief and fear associated with chronic illness diagnosis. Carmen learned to sit with Sofia's difficult emotions without immediately trying to fix or reframe them.

"Learning to say 'This is scary' instead of 'Everything will be fine' felt wrong at first," Carmen admits. "But Sofia started talking to me again when she realized I could handle her real feelings."

Managing Your Own Frustration

Family members experience legitimate frustrations when chronic illness affects their lives. Acknowledging and managing these feelings appropriately prevents them from damaging relationships or creating additional stress for everyone involved.

Sources of Family Frustration

Unpredictability creates ongoing stress for family members who struggle with the inability to plan or rely on consistent functioning from their loved one. Cancelled plans, modified activities, and last-minute changes challenge families who value predictability and routine.

Helplessness emerges when family members want to help but lack effective ways to improve their loved one's condition. The desire to fix or solve problems conflicts with the reality that these conditions require management rather than cures.

Lifestyle changes affect entire families, not just the diagnosed individual. Dietary restrictions, activity limitations, and social modifications impact everyone's experiences and choices.

Healthy Frustration Management Strategies

Acknowledging frustration as normal and understandable prevents guilt and shame from compounding the emotion. Family members aren't required to feel positive about chronic illness impacts—they're human beings dealing with challenging circumstances.

Finding appropriate outlets for frustration helps prevent it from affecting interactions with your loved one. This might include exercise, talking with friends, journaling, or seeking professional counseling support.

Distinguishing between frustration with the situation versus frustration with your loved one prevents misdirected emotions from damaging relationships. The illness creates the limitations, not your family member's choices or character.

Case Example 3: David's Frustration Management Journey

David's wife, Angela, developed severe MCAS that required significant lifestyle modifications for their entire family. Their active social life involving dinner parties and restaurant visits became impossible due to Angela's food triggers and chemical sensitivities.

"I was angry about losing our social life," David admits. "We had to stop hosting friends, couldn't try new restaurants, and Angela often felt too sick to attend events we'd planned. I felt like the illness was controlling our entire family."

Initially, David directed his frustration toward Angela, suggesting she wasn't trying hard enough to manage her triggers or that she was being overly cautious about food restrictions. This approach created conflict and increased Angela's isolation.

A support group for spouses of people with chronic illness helped David understand the difference between frustration with circumstances versus frustration with his wife. He learned strategies for managing his emotions while supporting Angela's medical needs.

"I realized I was grieving our old life while also learning to appreciate our new normal," David explains. "Accepting that these feelings were normal helped me find better ways to cope without taking it out on Angela."

Supporting Without Enabling

The line between helpful support and enabling dysfunction can blur when chronic illness affects family dynamics. Learning to support your loved one's autonomy while providing appropriate assistance requires ongoing calibration and communication.

Understanding the Support-Enabling Spectrum

Helpful support assists your loved one in maintaining their independence and managing their condition effectively. This might include helping with medication organization, providing transportation during symptom flares, or assisting with household tasks during particularly difficult periods.

Enabling behavior removes your loved one's responsibility for managing their own condition or makes decisions for them that they could make independently. This might include calling in sick for them without their request, avoiding all potential triggers without their input, or taking over all household responsibilities permanently.

The difference often lies in whether the support increases or decreases your loved one's sense of agency and capability over time. Healthy support builds confidence and independence, while enabling creates dependency and learned helplessness.

Practical Guidelines for Supportive Assistance

Asking before helping respects your loved one's autonomy and ensures your assistance is actually wanted. "Would it be helpful if I..." allows them to accept or decline support based on their current needs and preferences.

Collaborating on solutions rather than implementing your own ideas maintains your loved one's involvement in managing their condition. Working together on problem-solving builds skills and confidence rather than creating dependency.

Encouraging self-advocacy supports your loved one's ability to communicate their needs and boundaries effectively. This skill proves essential for medical appointments, workplace accommodations, and social situations.

Celebrating Small Victories

Chronic illness changes the scale of achievements and victories. Learning to recognize and celebrate progress within the context of ongoing challenges helps maintain hope and motivation for everyone involved.

Redefining Success and Achievement

Traditional achievement markers may no longer apply when chronic illness affects functioning. Graduating college, maintaining employment, or participating in social activities might represent enormous accomplishments for someone managing these conditions.

Daily functioning victories deserve recognition and celebration. Successfully managing a medication schedule, completing a grocery shopping trip, or attending a family event might represent significant achievements during difficult periods.

Progress often appears in subtle improvements rather than dramatic changes. Increased energy levels, improved sleep quality, or reduced symptom frequency might indicate meaningful progress even if overall functioning remains limited.

Creating Family Celebration Practices

Acknowledging small wins helps maintain positive momentum during long-term illness management. This might involve verbal recognition, special meals, or small rewards that mark progress and achievement.

Documenting progress through photos, journals, or family discussions helps everyone recognize improvement over time. Chronic illness can create a sense that nothing changes or improves, making progress documentation particularly valuable.

Including your loved one in defining what constitutes a victory ensures celebrations feel meaningful rather than patronizing. Their perspective on what represents progress guides appropriate recognition and support.

Building Emotional Resilience Together

Families that successfully support members with chronic invisible illness develop emotional resilience that benefits everyone involved. This resilience comes from practicing validation, managing frustration appropriately, supporting autonomy, and celebrating meaningful progress together.

The emotional skills required for supporting someone with chronic illness transfer to other family challenges and relationships. Learning to validate, listen without minimizing, and manage difficult emotions creates stronger family bonds overall.

Emotional support isn't a one-way street in families dealing with chronic illness. The person with the condition also provides support, love, and care to other family members, maintaining reciprocal relationships rather than purely caregiving dynamics.

Core Emotional Support Principles

- Validation acknowledges emotional experiences without requiring agreement or immediate solutions

- Listening without minimizing creates safety for authentic emotional expression
- Managing personal frustration appropriately prevents relationship damage
- Supporting autonomy while providing assistance maintains dignity and independence
- Celebrating small victories maintains hope and motivation during long-term challenges
- Emotional support skills benefit entire family systems, not just the person with chronic illness

Chapter 5: Advocacy and Communication

Your daughter sits across from the high school guidance counselor, explaining for the third time why she needs to use the elevator instead of climbing three flights of stairs between classes. The counselor's expression shifts between skepticism and confusion as she describes POTS symptoms—the invisible disability that makes her look perfectly healthy while her heart rate skyrockets with physical exertion.

Advocacy becomes a family skill set when invisible chronic illness enters your lives. Unlike visible disabilities that prompt immediate understanding and accommodation, POTS, MCAS, and EDS require constant education, explanation, and persistence to access appropriate support in medical, educational, workplace, and social settings (Shaw & McDaniel, 2020).

Medical Advocacy Strategies

Healthcare advocacy requires balancing respect for medical professionals with persistent pursuit of appropriate care. Many physicians receive limited training about these conditions, creating situations where families must educate providers while seeking treatment.

Preparing for Medical Appointments

Successful medical advocacy starts before entering the doctor's office. Organizing symptoms, treatment history, and specific questions maximizes limited appointment time and improves communication effectiveness.

Creating symptom logs with specific examples helps physicians understand the scope and impact of your loved one's condition. Vague descriptions like "feeling tired" carry less weight than detailed accounts: "heart rate increases from 72 to 145 within two minutes of standing, accompanied by dizziness and nausea."

Bringing research about these conditions to appointments can be helpful but requires diplomacy. Physicians may feel defensive if families appear to question their expertise, but many appreciate current research about conditions they rarely encounter in practice.

Advocating During Medical Visits

Family members can serve as witnesses and advocates during medical appointments, particularly when brain fog or anxiety affects your loved one's ability to communicate effectively. However, this role requires balance between support and taking over the conversation.

Asking for clarification ensures everyone understands treatment plans and recommendations. Medical professionals often use terminology that sounds clear to them but confuses patients and families. "Could you explain what that means in everyday terms?" prevents misunderstandings.

Requesting written instructions and treatment plans creates accountability and reference materials for future visits. Many treatment recommendations get forgotten or misunderstood without written documentation.

Case Example 1: Advocating for Proper POTS Diagnosis

Sixteen-year-old Marcus experienced months of fatigue, dizziness, and rapid heartbeat that his pediatrician attributed to "teenage stress" and "too much caffeine." His mother, Patricia, knew something more serious was happening but struggled to convince medical professionals to investigate further.

"I brought Marcus to the emergency room twice when his heart rate hit 160 just from walking to the bathroom," Patricia recalls. "Both times they said it was anxiety and sent us home with advice to reduce stress."

Patricia's advocacy breakthrough came when she found research about POTS and brought printed articles to Marcus's next appointment. She also documented his heart rate patterns using a home monitor, providing concrete evidence of orthostatic intolerance.

"Having numbers and research changed everything," Patricia explains. "The doctor could see the data and couldn't dismiss it as anxiety anymore. We got a referral to cardiology that same day."

Marcus received his POTS diagnosis three weeks later and began appropriate treatment. Patricia's persistent advocacy—backed by documentation and research—overcame initial medical dismissal and secured proper care.

School and Workplace Support

Educational and workplace advocacy requires understanding legal protections while building collaborative relationships with administrators and supervisors. The goal is creating environments where your loved one can succeed despite their medical limitations.

Educational Advocacy and Accommodations

Students with POTS, MCAS, and EDS qualify for accommodations under Section 504 plans or Individualized Education Programs (IEPs) depending on how their conditions affect educational access. These legal protections require specific documentation and advocacy to implement effectively.

Common educational accommodations include elevator access, extended time for assignments, modified physical education requirements, permission to leave class for medical needs, and alternative testing arrangements during symptom flares.

Building relationships with school personnel creates collaborative problem-solving opportunities. Teachers, counselors, and administrators who understand your student's conditions become allies in developing creative solutions to educational challenges.

Workplace Accommodation Strategies

Adult family members with these conditions benefit from understanding their rights under the Americans with Disabilities Act (ADA). Reasonable workplace accommodations can include flexible scheduling, modified duties, ergonomic equipment, and permission for medical appointments.

The accommodation request process requires medical documentation and clear communication about how specific limitations affect job performance. Vague requests for "help with fatigue" prove less effective than specific requests: "flexible start times to accommodate morning symptom management."

Successful workplace advocacy focuses on maintaining productivity while managing medical needs. Employers respond better to accommodation requests that demonstrate commitment to job performance rather than requests that seem to reduce accountability.

Case Example 2: Sarah's Workplace Accommodation Success

Sarah worked as a marketing coordinator when her MCAS symptoms began interfering with her job performance. Chemical sensitivities to office cleaning products and coworker perfumes triggered severe reactions that affected her concentration and attendance.

"I was calling in sick frequently and couldn't explain why the office environment was making me feel horrible," Sarah explains. "My supervisor thought I was having personal problems or wasn't committed to the job."

Sarah's husband helped her research ADA accommodation requirements and prepare a formal request. They worked with Sarah's doctor to document specific triggers and necessary accommodations, including fragrance-free workspace policies and air filtration equipment.

"The accommodation process took three months of back-and-forth communication," Sarah recalls. "But my employer ultimately provided an office with better ventilation and implemented a fragrance-free policy for my work area."

Sarah's job performance improved dramatically once her environmental triggers were addressed. Her supervisor became a strong advocate for accommodation policies that helped other employees with chemical sensitivities.

Extended Family Education

Extended family members often struggle to understand invisible chronic illness, creating tension during family gatherings and social events. Education and boundary-setting help manage these relationships while maintaining family connections.

Explaining Invisible Conditions to Family

Extended family education requires patience and repetition. Many relatives need multiple explanations before understanding how invisible conditions affect daily functioning. Providing written information supplements verbal explanations and gives family members time to process complex medical information.

Using analogies helps explain unfamiliar medical concepts. Describing POTS as "the body's circulation system not working properly" may be more understandable than detailed explanations of autonomic dysfunction.

Setting realistic expectations about improvement and recovery prevents family members from constantly asking about cures or dramatic improvement. Explaining that these are chronic conditions requiring ongoing management helps relatives understand why symptoms persist despite treatment.

Managing Family Judgment and Skepticism

Some family members struggle to accept invisible illness as legitimate, particularly when symptoms fluctuate or don't match their expectations of sickness. This skepticism can create painful family dynamics that require careful management.

Providing educational materials from reputable medical sources helps establish credibility for family members who question the legitimacy of these conditions. Information from organizations like the Dysautonomia International or Ehlers-Danlos Society carries more weight than family explanations.

Setting boundaries with unsupportive family members protects your loved one from harmful interactions while maintaining family relationships where possible. This might include limiting discussion of medical topics or avoiding certain family events during symptomatic periods.

Case Example 3: The Johnson Family Holiday Challenge

Every family holiday became a source of stress for the Johnson family after their daughter Emma was diagnosed with the trifecta. Emma's aunt consistently questioned why Emma needed to rest during family gatherings, suggesting she was being "antisocial" or "making excuses."

"Aunt Linda would make comments about Emma 'looking fine' and 'needing to push through,'" explains Emma's mother, Carol. "She'd compare Emma to other young people and suggest that Emma wasn't trying hard enough to participate."

The situation escalated during Christmas dinner when Linda publicly questioned Emma's need for dietary restrictions and suggested the family was "enabling" her behavior. Emma left the gathering in tears, and Carol realized direct intervention was necessary.

Carol sent Linda educational materials about MCAS and invited her to attend one of Emma's medical appointments. Linda's perspective shifted when she heard Emma's cardiologist explain the physiological basis for her symptoms and limitations.

"Seeing a doctor validate Emma's condition changed everything for Linda," Carol explains. "She became one of Emma's strongest advocates and helped educate other family members about invisible illness."

Friend Group Dynamics

Friendships face unique challenges when chronic invisible illness affects social activities and availability. Maintaining meaningful friendships requires communication about limitations while adapting social activities to accommodate medical needs.

Communicating with Friends About Limitations

Friends often lack understanding about chronic illness impacts on social functioning. They may interpret cancelled plans as lack of interest or assume that "looking good" means feeling well enough for activities.

Direct communication about specific limitations helps friends understand how to provide appropriate support. Explaining that "I have good days and bad days, and I might need to cancel plans last-minute" sets realistic expectations for social interactions.

Educating friends about your loved one's conditions helps them become allies rather than sources of pressure or misunderstanding. Friends who understand the unpredictable nature of symptoms become more flexible and supportive social partners.

Adapting Social Activities

Successful social adaptation involves modifying activities rather than eliminating them entirely. This might include shorter gatherings, seated activities, or events that accommodate dietary restrictions and environmental sensitivities.

Creating backup plans for social activities reduces stress when symptoms interfere with original plans. Having alternative options allows friendships to continue even when medical needs require modifications.

Encouraging friends to suggest inclusive activities helps maintain social connections while accommodating medical limitations. Friends who propose seated movie nights or low-key gatherings demonstrate understanding and support.

Public Situation Management

Public spaces present unique challenges for people with invisible chronic illness. Managing symptoms, accessing accommodations, and dealing with public misunderstanding requires preparation and confidence.

Accessing Public Accommodations

Disability parking permits benefit people with POTS and EDS who experience fatigue and mobility challenges, even if they don't always use mobility aids. These permits provide access to closer parking spaces that reduce walking distances during symptomatic periods.

Public restroom access becomes important for people managing MCAS symptoms or medication schedules. Knowing restroom locations and having emergency supplies readily available prevents complications during outings.

Airline accommodations include priority boarding, aisle seating, and permission to bring medical supplies. These accommodations require advance planning and medical documentation but significantly improve travel experiences.

Handling Public Misunderstanding

Public misunderstanding about invisible disability creates challenging social situations. Young people using disability parking or elevators may face criticism from others who don't understand invisible limitations.

Preparing responses to public comments helps your loved one manage these situations confidently. Simple explanations like "I have a medical condition that affects my mobility" often satisfy curious or critical observers.

Carrying medical identification cards or wearing medical alert jewelry provides credibility during emergencies or when accommodations are questioned. These visible indicators of medical conditions help validate accommodation needs.

Communication Excellence in Action

Effective advocacy requires persistence, preparation, and strategic communication across multiple environments. The skills developed through medical, educational, workplace, and social advocacy benefit your loved one throughout their lifetime while building family confidence in navigating complex systems.

The most successful advocacy efforts combine education with relationship-building. People respond better to advocacy efforts that teach them something new rather than demanding immediate compliance with requests they don't understand.

Advocacy becomes easier with practice and experience. Families develop confidence and expertise over time, becoming effective advocates not only for their loved one but for others facing similar challenges in various settings.

Advocacy Foundations for Success

- Medical advocacy requires preparation, documentation, and respectful persistence with healthcare providers
- Educational and workplace accommodations protect legal rights while building collaborative relationships
- Extended family education prevents misunderstanding and builds support networks
- Friend group communication maintains social connections while setting realistic expectations

- Public accommodation access requires confidence and preparation for challenging situations
- Effective advocacy combines education with relationship-building across all environments

Chapter 6: Redefining Family Roles

The family meeting convenes around the kitchen table on a Tuesday evening, but this isn't about vacation planning or household chores. Mom's POTS diagnosis has shifted everything—who drives to soccer practice, who manages dinner preparation, who handles the grocery shopping that once seemed so routine. The carefully constructed family ecosystem that operated smoothly for years now requires complete reorganization around invisible limitations and unpredictable symptoms.

Chronic invisible illness doesn't just affect the diagnosed individual—it reshapes entire family systems, forcing every member to adapt their roles, responsibilities, and expectations. The changes ripple through daily routines, long-term plans, and the fundamental ways family members relate to each other (Rolland, 2018).

When a Parent Is Ill

Parental illness with invisible chronic conditions creates unique challenges that differ significantly from temporary illnesses or visible disabilities. The parent may look perfectly healthy while struggling to maintain their traditional roles and responsibilities, creating confusion and adjustment difficulties for children and partners.

Shifting Parental Responsibilities

The active parent who coached little league and organized family adventures may need to step back from physically demanding activities. This doesn't mean becoming an inactive parent—it means redefining parental involvement around energy limitations and symptom fluctuations.

Cognitive symptoms like brain fog can affect a parent's ability to manage complex scheduling, financial decisions, or homework supervision. These invisible limitations require family adaptations that children may not initially understand or accept.

The disciplinary structure may need adjustment when a parent experiences chronic pain, fatigue, or other symptoms that affect their consistency and energy for enforcement. Maintaining parental authority while acknowledging limitations requires careful balance and communication.

Maintaining Parent-Child Relationships

Children need honest, age-appropriate explanations about their parent's condition to understand why family dynamics are changing. Hiding illness details often creates more anxiety and confusion than transparent communication about limitations and adaptations.

Quality time may need redefinition when physical limitations affect traditional parent-child activities. Reading together, working puzzles, or having conversations can become meaningful connection points when hiking or playing sports becomes impossible.

The parent's emotional availability remains crucial even when physical capacity decreases. Children benefit from understanding that their parent's love and interest haven't changed, even if their ability to participate in certain activities has shifted.

Case Example 1: Rebecca's Parenting Adaptation

Rebecca was diagnosed with the trifecta when her children were ages 8, 12, and 15. As a single mother who prided herself on being highly involved in her children's activities, the diagnosis forced major adjustments to her parenting approach.

"I used to volunteer for every field trip, attend every game, and host sleepovers regularly," Rebecca explains. "Suddenly, I could barely manage the grocery shopping without needing to rest for hours afterward."

Her oldest daughter, Sarah, initially reacted with anger and confusion when Rebecca began missing important events. "She thought I was choosing not to come rather than understanding that I physically couldn't handle the demands," Rebecca recalls.

The family worked with a counselor to develop new ways for Rebecca to show support and involvement. She became the team's unofficial photographer, taking pictures at games when she felt well enough to attend. She created elaborate care packages for field trips she couldn't chaperone and established traditions like post-game phone calls when attendance wasn't possible.

"My children learned that love and support come in many forms," Rebecca reflects. "I couldn't be the physically present parent I was before, but I found new ways to be emotionally available and supportive."

When a Child Is Ill

Childhood chronic invisible illness affects family roles differently than adult illness. Parents must balance protection with independence, advocacy with autonomy, and hope with realistic expectations about their child's capabilities and limitations.

Parental Role Adjustments

Parents often intensify their protective instincts when a child receives a chronic illness diagnosis. This protection can become counterproductive if it prevents the child from developing independence and self-advocacy skills necessary for managing their condition long-term.

The advocacy role expands significantly as parents navigate medical systems, educational accommodations, and social situations on behalf of a child who may not yet have the skills or confidence to self-advocate effectively.

Balancing the needs of the ill child with siblings requires careful attention and planning. The child with chronic illness may require more time, attention, and resources, creating potential resentment or feelings of neglect in healthy siblings.

Supporting Child Independence

Age-appropriate involvement in medical decision-making helps children develop ownership of their condition and builds skills they'll need as adults. This might include medication management, appointment scheduling, or communicating with healthcare providers.

Encouraging normal childhood activities within medical limitations prevents chronic illness from completely defining the child's identity and experiences. The goal is adaptation rather than avoidance of age-appropriate challenges and opportunities.

Teaching self-advocacy skills prepares children for adult independence while building confidence in their ability to manage their condition. These skills prove essential for educational settings, social situations, and future employment.

Case Example 2: Managing Emma's Teenage Years with MCAS

Emma developed severe MCAS symptoms at age 14, just as she was gaining independence and forming her identity separate from her family. Her parents, Janet and David, struggled with how much protection to provide versus encouraging normal teenage experiences.

"Emma wanted to go to sleepovers and eat at restaurants with friends, but we were terrified of anaphylactic reactions," Janet explains. "We felt torn between keeping her safe and letting her be a normal teenager."

The family developed a gradual independence plan that included Emma carrying emergency medications, learning to read ingredient labels carefully, and communicating with friends' parents about her dietary restrictions and emergency protocols.

"We started with shorter activities close to home and gradually increased Emma's independence as she demonstrated good judgment about managing her triggers," David recalls. "It was scary, but we realized that overprotection would leave her unprepared for adult life."

Emma learned to research restaurants before eating out, pack safe foods for events, and educate friends about her condition. These skills gave her confidence to participate in social activities while managing her medical needs responsibly.

Sibling Dynamics and Support

Siblings of children with chronic invisible illness face unique challenges that require attention and support. They may feel overlooked, confused about their sibling's limitations, or resentful about changes to family life and attention distribution.

Understanding Sibling Reactions

Healthy siblings often experience conflicting emotions about their brother or sister's illness. They may feel guilty for being healthy, angry about disrupted family plans, or confused about invisible symptoms that don't match their understanding of sickness.

The attention imbalance created by chronic illness management can lead to attention-seeking behaviors, academic problems, or emotional withdrawal in healthy siblings. These reactions are normal responses to family stress rather than character flaws.

Siblings may feel pressure to be "perfect" or avoid causing additional stress for parents who are already managing complex medical needs. This pressure can create anxiety and prevent healthy emotional expression.

Creating Sibling Support Systems

Open communication about the ill sibling's condition helps healthy siblings understand why family dynamics have changed. Age-appropriate explanations reduce confusion and resentment while building empathy and support.

Individual attention for healthy siblings ensures their needs don't get lost in the focus on medical management. This might include one-on-one time with parents, participation in their own activities, or support groups for siblings of chronically ill children.

Involving healthy siblings in age-appropriate ways can build family unity while giving them meaningful roles in supporting their brother or sister. This might include helping with medication reminders, attending medical appointments, or learning about the condition.

Case Example 3: The Wilson Family Sibling Dynamics

When 12-year-old Michael was diagnosed with EDS and POTS, his younger brother Jake initially seemed unaffected by the family changes. However, his parents soon noticed behavior changes including regression in potty training, difficulty sleeping, and increased clinginess.

"Jake was only 6, and he couldn't understand why Michael got to skip gym class, use the elevator at school, and receive extra attention for doctor appointments," explains their mother, Lisa. "He started having meltdowns and asking if he could be sick too."

The family implemented specific strategies to address Jake's needs while managing Michael's condition. They established weekly one-on-one time between Jake and each parent, created special activities that Jake could enjoy without Michael, and explained Michael's condition in terms Jake could understand.

"We told Jake that Michael's body works differently and needs extra help, just like how Jake needs glasses to see clearly," Lisa recalls. "We also made sure Jake had his own special activities and attention so he didn't feel forgotten."

The siblings eventually developed a supportive relationship where Jake became one of Michael's biggest advocates at school and in social situations, while maintaining his own identity and interests.

Spouse and Partner Adjustments

Marital and partnership relationships face significant challenges when chronic invisible illness affects one partner. The healthy partner often becomes a caregiver while grieving changes to their relationship and future plans.

Relationship Role Redistribution

Household responsibilities require redistribution based on the ill partner's capacity and limitations. This redistribution needs to be flexible, as energy and symptom levels fluctuate unpredictably with these conditions.

Financial responsibilities may shift if the ill partner's work capacity decreases or medical expenses increase. These changes can create stress and require ongoing communication about priorities and decision-making.

Social roles within the relationship may change as the ill partner's energy for social activities decreases. The healthy partner might attend events alone or the couple might need to find new ways to socialize that accommodate medical limitations.

Maintaining Intimacy and Connection

Physical intimacy often requires adaptation when chronic illness affects energy, pain levels, or comfort. Open communication about needs, limitations, and alternatives helps maintain physical connection despite medical challenges.

Emotional intimacy can strengthen through shared challenges, but it requires intentional effort to prevent caregiver-patient dynamics from replacing romantic partnership. Maintaining couple identity separate from illness management becomes crucial.

Shared activities may need modification but shouldn't be eliminated entirely. Finding new ways to connect and enjoy time together helps maintain relationship satisfaction despite chronic illness limitations.

Communication and Conflict Resolution

Chronic illness creates additional stressors that can increase relationship conflict. Learning to distinguish between illness-related stress and relationship problems helps couples address issues appropriately.

The healthy partner may experience caregiver fatigue, resentment about lifestyle changes, or fear about the future. These feelings are normal but need healthy expression and management to prevent relationship damage.

Regular relationship check-ins help couples stay connected and address problems before they become overwhelming. These conversations should focus on the relationship itself, not just illness management.

Extended Family Involvement

Extended family members can provide crucial support or create additional stress, depending on their understanding of invisible chronic illness and their approach to helping. Managing these relationships requires clear communication and boundary setting.

Educating Extended Family

Grandparents, aunts, uncles, and cousins often struggle to understand invisible chronic illness, particularly when symptoms fluctuate or don't match their expectations of sickness. Education helps build support while reducing judgment and unhelpful suggestions.

Extended family members may offer unsolicited advice about treatments, lifestyle changes, or alternative approaches. While well-intentioned, these suggestions can create stress and imply that current management approaches are inadequate.

Setting boundaries about medical discussions helps protect the family from constant questioning about treatments, progress, or future plans. Extended family members need to understand which topics are welcome and which create stress.

Building Extended Family Support

Extended family can provide practical support through childcare, meal preparation, transportation, or household help. This support becomes particularly valuable during symptom flares or medical crisis periods.

Emotional support from extended family helps combat the isolation often experienced by families dealing with chronic illness. Understanding relatives can provide encouragement, validation, and perspective during difficult periods.

Including extended family in appropriate ways helps maintain family relationships while managing chronic illness. This might include modified holiday celebrations, accessible family activities, or flexible visiting arrangements.

Approaching Change with Wisdom

Family role redefinition requires patience, flexibility, and ongoing communication as everyone adjusts to new realities. The process isn't linear—families may need to readjust roles multiple times as conditions change or new challenges emerge.

Successful families focus on maintaining core relationships and values while adapting practical arrangements to accommodate medical needs. The goal isn't returning to previous family dynamics but creating new patterns that work for everyone involved.

Role changes can strengthen family bonds by building empathy, cooperation, and resilience. Many families discover new strengths and closer relationships through the process of adapting to chronic illness challenges.

Building Blocks for Role Adaptation

- Parental illness requires honest communication and creative adaptations to maintain parent-child relationships
- Childhood chronic illness needs balanced protection with independence development and sibling support
- Sibling dynamics require attention to prevent resentment while building family unity and understanding
- Partnership relationships benefit from intentional intimacy maintenance and flexible responsibility distribution
- Extended family involvement requires education and boundary setting to maximize support while minimizing stress
- Successful role redefinition focuses on adaptation rather than returning to previous family patterns

Chapter 7: Financial and Practical Planning

The medical bills arrive in steady waves—copays for specialist appointments, costs for medications not covered by insurance, expenses for medical equipment that improves daily functioning but isn't considered "necessary" by insurance standards. Your kitchen table becomes a command center for insurance appeals, disability paperwork, and financial spreadsheets tracking medical expenses that seem to multiply faster than your ability to pay them.

Financial planning for families affected by POTS, MCAS, and EDS requires strategies that extend far beyond typical budgeting advice. These conditions create ongoing medical expenses, potential income loss, and the need for long-term financial security planning that accounts for chronic illness realities (Chen & Rizzo, 2019).

Medical Expense Management

Medical expenses for complex chronic conditions often exceed what families anticipate or budget for routine healthcare. The costs include obvious expenses like specialist visits and medications, but also hidden costs like travel to specialized care centers, adaptive equipment, and alternative treatments not covered by insurance.

Understanding the Full Cost Structure

Direct medical costs include specialist copays, which can range from 50 to 200 dollars per visit for out-of-network providers. Many people with these conditions see multiple specialists regularly—cardiologists, gastroenterologists, neurologists, and pain management physicians—creating substantial monthly copay expenses.

Medication costs vary significantly based on insurance coverage and the specific drugs prescribed. Some POTS medications are available generically and cost relatively little, while MCAS medications might include expensive specialty drugs or require compounding pharmacies that charge premium prices.

Diagnostic testing expenses accumulate quickly during the diagnostic process and ongoing monitoring. Tilt table tests, autonomic testing, and specialized laboratory work often carry high costs, particularly when performed at specialized centers.

Hidden and Indirect Costs

Travel expenses become significant when specialized care requires trips to distant medical centers. Many patients with these conditions need to travel hundreds of miles to access knowledgeable physicians, creating costs for gas, hotels, meals, and lost work time.

Home modifications and adaptive equipment improve quality of life but rarely qualify for insurance coverage. Compression stockings, shower chairs, ergonomic furniture, and air purification systems represent ongoing expenses that add up over time.

Lost income affects many families when chronic illness reduces work capacity or requires frequent medical appointments. Even when disability benefits are available, they typically replace only a portion of previous income.

Case Example 1: The Martinez Family's Medical Expense Reality

Rosa Martinez's diagnosis with the trifecta created medical expenses that quickly overwhelmed the family's budget. Her husband Carlos worked as a teacher, and their insurance covered basic medical needs but not the specialized care Rosa required.

"The first year after diagnosis, we spent over $15,000 out of pocket on medical expenses," Carlos explains. "Rosa needed to see specialists in three different cities, none of whom were in our insurance network. The copays alone were over $300 per month."

The family's expenses included monthly visits to an out-of-network cardiologist, quarterly trips to a MCAS specialist 200 miles away, medications that cost $400 monthly after insurance, and adaptive equipment like compression stockings and a shower chair.

"We had to use credit cards for medical expenses and eventually took a second mortgage on our house," Carlos recalls. "We never anticipated how expensive it would be to get proper care for conditions most doctors don't understand."

The Martinez family learned to track all medical expenses meticulously for tax deduction purposes and began setting aside money in a health savings account to prepare for ongoing costs.

Insurance Navigation Together

Insurance systems often prove inadequate for managing complex chronic conditions that require specialized care and treatments. Families must learn to advocate effectively within insurance systems while understanding their rights and options for appeals and coverage.

Understanding Coverage Limitations

Many insurance plans limit coverage for out-of-network specialists, creating challenges when local physicians lack expertise in these conditions. Patients may need to choose between receiving appropriate care and managing costs within their insurance network.

Prior authorization requirements can delay necessary treatments and create administrative burdens for families already managing complex medical needs. Understanding these processes helps families prepare for delays and advocate more effectively.

Coverage for adaptive equipment and home modifications varies significantly between insurance plans. Many plans consider these items "convenience" rather than medical necessities, leaving families to pay out of pocket for items that significantly improve quality of life.

Effective Insurance Advocacy Strategies

Documentation becomes crucial for insurance appeals and coverage requests. Maintaining detailed records of symptoms, treatments tried, and medical necessity helps support requests for coverage of specialized care or equipment.

Understanding appeals processes allows families to challenge coverage denials effectively. Many insurance denials are overturned on appeal when families provide appropriate documentation and persist through the process.

Working with healthcare providers to support insurance requests improves success rates for coverage appeals. Physicians familiar with insurance requirements can provide documentation that meets specific criteria for coverage approval.

Case Example 2: Navigating Insurance for Emma's MCAS Treatment

Emma's MCAS required medications that her insurance initially refused to cover, classifying them as "experimental" despite their effectiveness for her symptoms. Her mother, Jennifer, had to learn insurance advocacy quickly to access necessary treatments.

"The insurance company denied coverage for Emma's mast cell stabilizer medication three times," Jennifer explains. "Each denial letter said the medication wasn't approved for her diagnosis, even though her allergist explained it was standard treatment."

Jennifer learned to submit appeals with supporting documentation from Emma's physician, research studies about MCAS treatment, and detailed records of Emma's symptom improvement with the medication. The appeal process took six months and multiple submissions.

"I spent hours on the phone with insurance representatives, learning their internal processes and requirements," Jennifer recalls. "Eventually, we got coverage approved, but it required persistence and detailed documentation."

The family also learned to purchase medications in three-month supplies when possible to reduce copay costs and avoid frequent prior authorization renewals.

Disability Application Support

Disability applications for invisible chronic illness require extensive documentation and often face initial denials. Family support during this process proves crucial for gathering necessary information and maintaining persistence through appeals.

Understanding Disability Criteria

Social Security Disability evaluates functional limitations rather than just diagnoses. The application must demonstrate how symptoms prevent the ability to work consistently, not just during occasional flares.

The "listing" approach compares applicant conditions to specific criteria in Social Security's Blue Book. However, POTS, MCAS, and EDS don't have specific listings, requiring applications to demonstrate equivalence to related conditions.

Residual Functional Capacity assessments evaluate what work activities someone can perform despite their limitations. This evaluation considers physical capacity, cognitive function, and the ability to maintain consistent attendance and performance.

Building Strong Disability Applications

Medical documentation from specialists familiar with these conditions carries more weight than general practitioner records. Specialists can provide detailed explanations of how symptoms affect daily functioning and work capacity.

Functional assessments document specific limitations in standing, walking, lifting, concentrating, and maintaining consistent energy levels. Objective testing results support subjective symptom reports.

Work history documentation shows previous employment success and demonstrates that current limitations represent a change from normal capacity rather than a long-term pattern of work avoidance.

Case Example 3: David's Disability Application Journey

David worked as an accountant before developing severe POTS that made maintaining consistent work impossible. His disability application process took three years and required extensive family support to gather necessary documentation.

"David's cognitive symptoms made it impossible for him to manage the paperwork and appointments required for the disability application," explains his wife, Sarah. "I had to become his advocate and organize all the medical records and documentation."

The initial application was denied because the reviewer didn't understand how POTS affects work capacity. The appeal required additional medical testing, detailed physician reports, and documentation of David's work limitations.

"We had to prove that David couldn't work consistently, not just that he had POTS," Sarah explains. "This required showing how his symptoms affected his concentration, energy levels, and ability to sit or stand for extended periods."

David's disability approval came after demonstrating that his condition prevented him from maintaining any consistent work schedule, even with accommodations. The process required family support throughout due to his cognitive limitations during the application period.

Estate Planning Considerations

Chronic illness creates estate planning needs that differ from standard financial planning. Families must consider scenarios where the ill person's condition worsens, where medical expenses exhaust family resources, or where premature death occurs.

Special Needs Trust Considerations

Special needs trusts protect assets while maintaining eligibility for government benefits. These trusts can supplement disability income without jeopardizing benefit eligibility.

Asset protection becomes important when medical expenses threaten family financial security. Proper estate planning can protect assets from medical creditors while ensuring continued care access.

Family coordination ensures that extended family members understand estate planning decisions and their roles in supporting the chronically ill family member if needed.

Healthcare Directive Planning

Healthcare proxies need specific instructions about treatment preferences during medical emergencies or periods when cognitive symptoms prevent decision-making. Standard healthcare directives may not address the complexity of chronic illness management.

Medical information organization helps healthcare proxies make informed decisions during emergencies. This includes current medication lists, specialist contact information, and treatment preferences.

Financial power of attorney documents allow trusted family members to manage medical expenses and insurance issues during periods when the ill person cannot handle these responsibilities independently.

Emergency Planning

Medical emergencies take on different characteristics when chronic illness is involved. Emergency planning must account for baseline medical complexity, medication requirements, and the need for specialized care that may not be available in standard emergency settings.

Medical Emergency Preparedness

Emergency medical information cards should include current medications, known triggers, emergency contacts, and specific instructions for healthcare providers unfamiliar with these conditions. This information proves crucial during emergency situations when the patient may not be able to communicate effectively.

Emergency medication supplies need to be maintained and easily accessible. This includes rescue medications for MCAS reactions, emergency hydration supplies for POTS, and pain management medications for EDS flares.

Hospital communication plans help ensure that emergency medical providers understand the complexity of these conditions and avoid treatments that might worsen symptoms. Many standard emergency treatments can be problematic for people with MCAS or POTS.

Financial Emergency Planning

Emergency funds specifically for medical crises help families manage unexpected medical expenses without depleting general emergency savings. These funds should be separate from routine medical expense budgets.

Insurance emergency procedures include understanding how to access out-of-network emergency care and the steps required for emergency authorization of treatments or medications.

Family financial coordination ensures that someone can manage medical expenses and insurance issues if the primary financial manager becomes incapacitated due to medical emergency or symptom flare.

Planning for Sustainable Security

The most effective financial planning for families affected by chronic illness balances current medical needs with long-term financial security. This requires realistic assessment of ongoing costs while building systems that provide stability during medical and financial crises.

Successful financial management combines careful budgeting with strategic advocacy to maximize insurance benefits and minimize out-of-pocket expenses. Families who invest time in understanding insurance systems and disability processes often achieve better financial outcomes.

Financial planning for chronic illness requires flexibility and ongoing adjustment as medical needs change over time. The strategies that work during stable periods may need modification during symptom progression or improvement.

Building Blocks for Financial Security

- Medical expense management requires understanding both direct and hidden costs of chronic illness care
- Insurance navigation benefits from persistent advocacy and detailed documentation of medical necessity
- Disability applications need specialist documentation and family support throughout the complex process
- Estate planning must account for chronic illness scenarios and protection of assets from medical expenses
- Emergency planning includes both medical and financial preparations for crisis situations
- Successful financial management balances current needs with long-term security through flexible planning approaches

Chapter 8: Preventing Caregiver Burnout

The alarm clock screams at 5:30 AM, but you've been awake for an hour already, your mind racing through today's medical appointments, medication schedules, and the growing stack of insurance appeals on your kitchen counter. Your coffee tastes bitter as you review the day's caregiving tasks while your loved one sleeps peacefully, unaware that you've spent another sleepless night worrying about their condition—and your own ability to keep managing everything.

Caregiver burnout creeps up slowly, disguising itself as dedication and love until exhaustion becomes your constant companion. The statistics paint a sobering picture: family caregivers experience depression at twice the rate of non-caregivers, and 40 to 70 percent show signs of clinical depression within the first year of caregiving (Schulz & Sherwood, 2008). These numbers aren't just statistics—they represent real families struggling to balance love with self-preservation.

Recognizing Burnout Signs

Caregiver burnout manifests differently from typical stress or fatigue. It develops gradually, often masked by the belief that exhaustion and overwhelm are normal parts of caring for someone with chronic illness. Understanding the specific signs of burnout helps distinguish between temporary stress and serious emotional depletion that requires immediate attention.

Physical Manifestations of Burnout

Chronic fatigue that doesn't improve with rest becomes a hallmark of caregiver burnout. This exhaustion differs from normal tiredness—it penetrates your bones and makes simple tasks feel monumental. You might find yourself struggling to get out of bed despite sleeping poorly, or falling asleep during conversations.

Sleep disturbances plague burned-out caregivers, creating a vicious cycle where worry prevents rest, and lack of rest reduces your ability to cope with stress. You might lie awake planning tomorrow's caregiving tasks or wake up multiple times checking on your loved one unnecessarily.

Physical symptoms often mirror those experienced by the person you're caring for. Headaches, digestive issues, muscle tension, and frequent illnesses signal that your body is overwhelmed by chronic stress. Your immune system weakens under sustained pressure, making you more susceptible to every virus that circulates through your community.

Emotional and Cognitive Warning Signs

Irritability becomes your default response to minor inconveniences or requests. You might snap at family members, feel annoyed by your loved one's needs, or react disproportionately to small problems. This irritability often comes with guilt, creating an emotional spiral that compounds your distress.

Brain fog—the same cognitive symptom your loved one experiences—can affect caregivers under chronic stress. You might forget appointments, struggle to make decisions, or find yourself unable to concentrate on conversations or tasks that once came easily.

Emotional numbness serves as a protective mechanism when feelings become too overwhelming to process. You might notice that activities you once enjoyed feel meaningless, or that you're going through the motions of caregiving without feeling connected to the purpose behind your actions.

Case Example 1: Recognizing Sarah's Caregiver Burnout

Sarah had been caring for her husband Mark through his POTS and MCAS diagnosis for two years when her adult daughter visited for the holidays. Within hours of arrival, her daughter noticed changes that Sarah hadn't recognized in herself.

"Mom was snapping at Dad for every little thing—asking for water, needing help getting dressed, wanting to rest," recalls their daughter, Jessica. "She looked exhausted, and she'd forgotten several important appointments that week."

Sarah had been experiencing insomnia for months, lying awake worrying about Mark's symptoms and planning the next day's medical tasks. She'd stopped reading, given up her weekly coffee dates with friends, and hadn't realized she'd lost fifteen pounds from skipping meals while focused on Mark's dietary needs.

"I thought I was just being a good wife," Sarah explains. "I didn't realize that my exhaustion and irritability meant I was actually becoming less helpful to Mark and more stressed myself."

Jessica's outside perspective helped Sarah recognize that her dedication had crossed into burnout territory. The family arranged for additional support so Sarah could begin addressing her own physical and emotional depletion.

Setting Sustainable Boundaries

Boundary setting in caregiving relationships requires delicate balance between providing necessary support and maintaining your own well-being. Many caregivers struggle with guilt when establishing limits, but sustainable boundaries actually improve your ability to provide quality care over the long term.

Distinguishing Between Needs and Wants

Your loved one has legitimate medical needs that require assistance—medication management during brain fog episodes, transportation to medical appointments, or help during severe symptom flares. These needs differ from preferences or conveniences that, while understandable, don't require your immediate response.

Learning to distinguish between urgent medical needs and requests that can wait helps prevent the constant state of alert that exhausts caregivers. Your loved one might prefer that you handle all meal preparation, but they may be capable of managing simple meals during stable periods.

The goal isn't to become less helpful but to focus your energy on situations where your assistance is truly necessary. This approach preserves your capacity for genuine emergencies while encouraging your loved one's independence in areas where they can function safely.

Creating Physical and Time Boundaries

Establishing specific caregiving hours helps prevent the around-the-clock vigilance that leads to burnout. Unless your loved one requires constant supervision for safety reasons, you need time when you're not responsible for monitoring their symptoms or needs.

Physical space boundaries matter even in close relationships. Your loved one's bedroom doesn't need to become your secondary office for medical record management. Creating separate spaces for caregiving tasks and personal time helps maintain psychological boundaries.

Sleep protection becomes non-negotiable for caregiver health. This might mean using baby monitors instead of sleeping in the same room, establishing quiet hours when non-emergency needs wait until morning, or arranging overnight help during particularly difficult periods.

Communication Strategies for Boundary Setting

Explaining boundaries in terms of long-term caregiving sustainability helps your loved one understand that limits protect your ability to provide ongoing support. "I need to maintain my health so I can continue helping you effectively" frames boundaries as caregiving strategy rather than selfishness.

Collaborative boundary setting involves your loved one in establishing reasonable limits and backup plans for times when you're not available. This approach maintains their dignity while ensuring their needs are met through multiple sources rather than relying solely on you.

Regular boundary reviews allow adjustments as your loved one's condition changes or as you identify areas where boundaries need strengthening or relaxing. Flexibility in boundary implementation prevents rigid rules that don't serve anyone's best interests.

Case Example 2: The Johnson Family's Boundary Success

When their teenage son Michael was diagnosed with EDS, his parents Linda and Robert initially committed to 24-hour availability for any needs or concerns. Within six months, both parents were exhausted, their marriage was strained, and Michael had become overly dependent on their assistance.

"Michael would wake us up three or four times a night to help him reposition because of joint pain," Linda explains. "We were getting two or three hours of sleep, and during the day we were doing everything for him that he asked for."

The family worked with a therapist to establish sustainable boundaries that met Michael's legitimate needs while protecting his parents' well-being. They established quiet hours from 10 PM to 7 AM when Michael would use pain management techniques independently unless experiencing a genuine emergency.

"We set up his room with everything he might need during the night—extra pillows, heating pads, pain medication, and water," Robert explains. "We also taught him some positioning techniques he could do independently."

The boundary setting initially created some resistance from Michael, who had become accustomed to immediate parental response to every discomfort. However, the changes ultimately improved the entire family's functioning and Michael's confidence in managing his condition independently.

Building Support Networks

Isolation compounds caregiver stress and reduces your access to practical help and emotional support. Building networks requires intentional effort, but the investment pays dividends in reduced stress and increased caregiving sustainability.

Professional Support Systems

Healthcare teams can provide more than medical treatment—they can offer guidance on caregiving strategies, resources for respite care, and realistic expectations about your loved one's needs and capabilities. Don't hesitate to ask medical professionals about caregiver support resources.

Mental health professionals who understand chronic illness can help you process the complex emotions of caregiving while developing strategies for stress management and relationship preservation. Many therapists offer support groups specifically for chronic illness families.

Social workers connected to medical centers or community organizations can help you access practical resources like respite care, financial assistance programs, or adaptive equipment that reduces caregiving demands.

Family and Friend Networks

Extended family members often want to help but don't know how to contribute meaningfully. Creating specific volunteer opportunities—grocery shopping, transportation to appointments, or staying with your loved one during respite periods—channels their good intentions into practical support.

Friend networks require honesty about your caregiving challenges and specific requests for help. Many friends feel uncomfortable offering assistance because they don't understand chronic illness or worry about saying the wrong thing. Direct communication about your needs helps them provide appropriate support.

Caregiver support groups, both online and in-person, connect you with others who understand the unique challenges of caring for someone with invisible chronic illness. These connections provide emotional validation and practical advice from people with similar experiences.

Case Example 3: Building Maria's Support Network

Maria felt completely isolated while caring for her daughter Elena, who had been diagnosed with the trifecta during her senior year of high school. Maria's husband worked long hours, extended family lived far away, and she had gradually withdrawn from friendships due to caregiving demands.

"I felt like nobody understood what we were going through," Maria explains. "Elena looked fine to everyone else, so people would make comments about her being lucky to 'get out of' normal activities, not realizing how sick she actually was."

Maria's breakthrough came when Elena's cardiologist referred them to a support group for families dealing with dysautonomia. Meeting other parents who understood the challenges of invisible chronic illness provided immediate emotional relief and practical advice.

"The other parents shared strategies I'd never thought of, like how to handle school accommodations and which specialists were most helpful," Maria recalls. "But just as important was the feeling that I wasn't crazy or overprotective—other families were dealing with the same challenges."

Maria also reconnected with two close friends, explaining Elena's condition and asking for specific help with grocery shopping and transportation. Both friends appreciated understanding how they could help and became regular sources of practical and emotional support.

Respite Care Strategies

Respite care provides temporary relief from caregiving responsibilities, allowing you to rest, attend to personal needs, or simply have time away from medical concerns. Effective respite care requires planning and often involves multiple people or resources.

Informal Respite Options

Family members can provide respite care when properly educated about your loved one's condition and needs. This education includes understanding medication schedules, recognizing concerning symptoms, and knowing when to call for emergency help.

Friend networks can offer respite for specific activities—staying with your loved one while you attend medical appointments for yourself, providing transportation for routine errands, or simply offering companionship that doesn't require your presence.

Reciprocal arrangements with other caregiving families create mutual support systems where families take turns providing respite care. These arrangements work particularly well when children have similar conditions and families understand each other's challenges.

Professional Respite Services

Home health aides trained in chronic illness care can provide respite ranging from a few hours to several days. These professionals understand medical needs while allowing you to leave home with confidence that your loved one is safe and well-cared for.

Adult day programs designed for people with chronic illness offer socialization and supervision while giving caregivers extended respite periods. These programs often include medical monitoring and therapeutic activities.

Respite care facilities provide overnight or weekend relief for caregivers who need extended time away. These facilities specialize in caring for people with complex medical needs in supportive environments.

Planning Effective Respite

Preparation for respite care includes creating detailed instruction sheets about medication schedules, emergency procedures, preferred comfort measures, and contact information for medical providers. This preparation ensures continuity of care and reduces your anxiety while away.

Gradual introduction of respite providers helps your loved one become comfortable with new caregivers and allows you to assess the quality of care provided. Start with short periods and increase duration as comfort levels improve.

Regular respite scheduling prevents burnout by ensuring you have consistent breaks from caregiving responsibilities. Weekly or monthly respite periods provide something to look forward to and help maintain your emotional and physical health.

Maintaining Your Identity

Chronic caregiving can consume your identity until you forget who you were before illness entered your family. Maintaining connections to your individual interests, relationships, and goals preserves your sense of self and ultimately makes you a more effective caregiver.

Preserving Personal Interests

Hobbies and interests require adaptation rather than abandonment during intensive caregiving periods. You might need to modify how you engage in activities you enjoy, but maintaining some connection to personal interests preserves mental health and personal identity.

Creative outlets provide emotional release and cognitive stimulation that counterbalance the stress of caregiving. Writing, art, music, or crafts offer ways to process emotions while creating something meaningful for yourself.

Physical activities adapted to your available time and energy help manage caregiver stress while maintaining your health. This might include brief walks, yoga videos, or online fitness classes that fit around caregiving schedules.

Professional and Educational Pursuits

Career considerations require honest assessment of your caregiving demands and professional goals. Some caregivers find that reduced work hours or flexible arrangements allow them to maintain professional identity while meeting caregiving responsibilities.

Educational opportunities, including online courses or workshops related to chronic illness, can provide personal growth while building skills that benefit your caregiving role. Learning new information helps maintain cognitive engagement and sense of purpose.

Volunteer activities connected to chronic illness advocacy or support can channel your caregiving experience into meaningful community contribution while connecting you with others who share similar experiences.

Relationship Maintenance Outside Caregiving

Friendships require intentional nurturing during intensive caregiving periods. This might mean shorter visits, phone conversations instead of in-person meetings, or activities that can include your loved one when appropriate.

Couple relationships need attention separate from caregiving dynamics. Partners benefit from spending time together that isn't focused on medical needs or caregiving tasks. Professional counseling can help couples maintain connection during stressful periods.

Family relationships with siblings, parents, or children not directly involved in caregiving provide perspectives and connections that exist outside the medical context. These relationships remind you of your identity beyond caregiving.

The Path to Sustainable Caregiving

Preventing caregiver burnout requires ongoing attention to your own needs while providing appropriate support to your loved one. The goal isn't perfect balance—it's sustainable practices that allow you to maintain your health and relationships while providing quality care over the long term.

Recognition that caregiver burnout helps no one provides permission to prioritize your own well-being. A burned-out caregiver becomes less effective at providing support and may develop health problems that require additional family resources.

Building systems that support both you and your loved one creates resilience for your entire family. These systems evolve as conditions change, but the foundation of mutual support and realistic expectations provides stability during difficult periods.

Burnout Prevention Essentials

- Burnout recognition includes physical exhaustion, emotional numbness, and cognitive difficulties that don't improve with rest
- Sustainable boundaries distinguish between medical needs and preferences while protecting caregiver capacity
- Support networks require intentional building and maintenance but provide essential practical and emotional assistance
- Respite care planning ensures regular breaks from caregiving responsibilities through family, friends, or professional services
- Identity maintenance involves preserving personal interests, relationships, and goals separate from caregiving roles
- Sustainable caregiving benefits both caregiver and care recipient through improved health and relationship quality

Chapter 9: Relationship Preservation

The photograph on your nightstand shows you and your partner laughing at a restaurant, arms around each other without a care in the world. That picture feels like it was taken in another lifetime—before POTS changed your energy levels, before MCAS restricted your dining options, before EDS made physical intimacy complicated and sometimes painful. You love your partner deeply, but the relationship you once shared seems buried under medication schedules, doctor appointments, and the constant management of invisible symptoms.

Chronic illness doesn't just affect individuals—it reshapes every relationship within its reach, demanding adaptations that can either strengthen bonds or strain them to the breaking point. Research indicates that couples dealing with chronic illness face divorce rates 75% higher than healthy couples, yet many relationships not only survive but thrive when partners learn to adapt together (Revenson et al., 2016).

Intimacy and Chronic Illness

Physical intimacy becomes complex when chronic illness affects energy, comfort, and predictability. The spontaneous physical connection that many couples take for granted requires planning, adaptation, and open communication about changing needs and limitations.

Redefining Physical Intimacy

Traditional concepts of physical intimacy may need complete reconstruction when chronic illness affects energy levels, joint stability, or autonomic function. What once felt natural and effortless might now require careful positioning, timing around symptoms, and awareness of medication effects.

Pain and fatigue create real barriers to physical intimacy, but they don't eliminate the possibility of meaningful physical connection.

Many couples discover that slower, gentler approaches to intimacy become more satisfying than their previous patterns once they adjust expectations and communication.

POTS symptoms like rapid heart rate, dizziness, and fatigue during physical exertion require modifications to intimate activities. Partners learn to recognize when symptoms are manageable versus when physical intimacy should be postponed for health reasons.

Emotional Intimacy During Medical Challenges

Emotional intimacy often deepens during chronic illness as couples navigate challenges together and develop new forms of vulnerability and support. Sharing fears about the future, discussing treatment options, and supporting each other through difficult days can strengthen emotional bonds.

Communication about needs becomes more explicit when physical limitations affect relationship dynamics. Partners who previously relied on non-verbal cues or assumptions must learn to articulate their emotional and physical needs clearly.

The fear of being a burden can create emotional distance if the ill partner withdraws to protect their spouse from additional stress. Open discussion about these fears helps couples address concerns directly rather than letting assumptions damage their connection.

Case Example 1: Rebuilding Intimacy for Tom and Jennifer

Tom and Jennifer had been married for eight years when Jennifer's MCAS and EDS symptoms began affecting their physical relationship. Chemical sensitivities made Jennifer reactive to Tom's cologne and shampoo, while joint pain made their usual physical intimacy uncomfortable and sometimes impossible.

"I felt like I was constantly rejecting Tom," Jennifer explains. "I wanted to be close to him, but my body wouldn't cooperate. I was afraid he'd eventually get tired of dealing with my limitations and find someone without all these problems."

Tom initially interpreted Jennifer's physical withdrawal as emotional rejection, creating tension and misunderstanding between them. Both partners felt frustrated and disconnected, but neither knew how to address the changes without causing hurt feelings.

The couple worked with a counselor who specialized in chronic illness relationships to develop new approaches to intimacy. They created a fragrance-free bedroom environment, experimented with different timing around Jennifer's symptom cycles, and found new ways to connect physically that accommodated her joint limitations.

"We learned that intimacy isn't just about one specific activity," Tom reflects. "We discovered new ways to be close that actually brought us closer together than we'd been before Jennifer got sick."

Maintaining Friendship Within Caregiving

The balance between romantic partnership and caregiver relationship requires careful attention to prevent medical management from overwhelming the friendship and companionship that form the foundation of strong relationships.

Preserving Non-Medical Conversations

Chronic illness can dominate couple conversations until every interaction revolves around symptoms, treatments, or medical appointments. Intentionally creating space for non-medical discussions helps maintain the intellectual and emotional connection that exists beyond illness management.

Establishing "medical-free" times or zones in your home provides opportunities to discuss books, current events, shared interests, or future dreams without the weight of health concerns. These conversations remind couples of their connection beyond illness management.

The ill partner particularly needs opportunities to be seen as a whole person rather than a collection of symptoms requiring management. Discussing their thoughts, opinions, and interests unrelated to health helps maintain their sense of identity within the relationship.

Shared Activities and Interests

Activities may require modification but shouldn't be eliminated entirely. Couples who enjoyed hiking together might discover that nature photography or bird watching provides similar outdoor connection with less physical demand.

New shared interests can develop around the adaptations required by chronic illness. Some couples become advocates together, travel to medical conferences, or develop expertise in nutrition and wellness that becomes a shared passion.

The key is finding activities that both partners can enjoy rather than the ill partner participating out of obligation or the healthy partner sacrificing all their interests. Compromise and creativity help couples discover new ways to spend meaningful time together.

Case Example 2: The Peterson Family's Activity Adaptation

Mark and Lisa Peterson were avid travelers who had visited twenty-three countries together before Mark's severe POTS symptoms made their travel style impossible. Their relationship had been built around shared adventures and exploration, and both partners struggled with the loss of this central connection.

"Travel was our thing," Lisa explains. "We planned trips constantly, saved money for adventures, and defined ourselves as explorers. When Mark became too sick to travel, I felt like we'd lost the foundation of our relationship."

Mark felt guilty about limiting Lisa's opportunities for adventure while also grieving the loss of experiences that had brought him joy and purpose. The couple initially tried to maintain their previous travel patterns, resulting in several disastrous trips that left Mark severely symptomatic and both partners frustrated.

They eventually developed new approaches to exploration that accommodated Mark's limitations. They began taking shorter trips to nearby destinations, staying in accommodations with medical facilities nearby, and planning itineraries around Mark's energy patterns rather than tourist schedules.

"We also started exploring our own area more thoroughly," Mark adds. "We discovered museums, gardens, and historical sites within an hour of home that we'd never visited. Our adventures became smaller scale but more intimate."

Date Nights and Connection

Regular couple time away from medical concerns becomes more challenging but also more important when chronic illness affects daily life. Creating opportunities for romance and fun requires intentional planning and creative adaptation.

Planning Around Symptom Patterns

Successful date planning requires understanding your partner's symptom patterns and energy cycles. Some people with POTS feel better in the morning, while others have more energy in the evening. MCAS symptoms might be triggered by certain environments or foods, requiring careful venue selection.

Flexibility becomes essential for date planning because symptom flares can disrupt the best-laid plans. Having backup options—perhaps a quiet dinner at home instead of a restaurant, or a movie night instead of a concert—prevents disappointment and maintains connection even when symptoms interfere.

The definition of "date night" may need expansion to include activities that accommodate energy limitations. A meaningful conversation over coffee might replace dinner and dancing, but the intention to connect romantically remains the same.

Creating Romance Within Limitations

Romance adapts to new circumstances rather than disappearing entirely. Surprise gifts might shift from elaborate gestures to thoughtful accommodations like a new pillow for better sleep or a favorite meal delivered during a difficult symptom day.

Home-based dates become more frequent and often more intimate than public activities. Cooking together, having wine tastings, or creating spa experiences at home provide romantic connection without the energy demands of going out.

The effort invested in adaptation often increases the meaning of romantic gestures. When simple activities require planning and accommodation, the thoughtfulness involved demonstrates deep care and commitment.

Case Example 3: Recreating Romance for David and Sarah

David and Sarah had established weekly date nights during their five-year marriage, but Sarah's MCAS symptoms made restaurant dining nearly impossible due to food triggers and chemical sensitivities. Their previous romantic routine of trying new restaurants and attending live entertainment became sources of stress rather than connection.

"Every restaurant became a potential disaster," Sarah explains. "I'd spend the entire evening worried about having a reaction, and David would be watching me for symptoms instead of enjoying our time together."

The couple initially tried to maintain their restaurant routine by researching menus and calling ahead about ingredients, but the stress and frequent symptom reactions made dining out unenjoyable for both partners.

They eventually created elaborate home date nights that became more romantic and intimate than their previous restaurant outings. David learned to cook Sarah's safe foods creatively, they set up candlelit dinners in their backyard, and they discovered online entertainment options like virtual museum tours and live-streamed concerts.

"Our dates became more personal and thoughtful," David reflects. "Instead of relying on restaurants and venues to create romance, we had to be creative and intentional about connecting with each other."

Managing Resentment

Resentment can build slowly in relationships affected by chronic illness as both partners struggle with losses, limitations, and lifestyle changes. Addressing resentment openly and honestly prevents it from damaging the fundamental love and respect that hold relationships together.

Recognizing Sources of Resentment

The healthy partner may experience resentment about lifestyle limitations, increased responsibilities, or the loss of future plans they had envisioned. These feelings create guilt because they seem selfish when compared to their partner's suffering, but suppressing them allows resentment to grow.

The ill partner might resent their dependence on their spouse, the loss of their previous capabilities, or the feeling that they're a burden rather than an equal partner. They may also resent their partner's health and continued ability to engage in activities that are no longer possible for them.

Both partners might resent the illness itself and its impact on their relationship, but directing that resentment toward each other becomes easier than facing the uncertainty and unfairness of chronic illness.

Healthy Expression of Difficult Emotions

Professional counseling provides a safe space for both partners to express resentment, fear, and grief without damaging their relationship. A therapist familiar with chronic illness can help couples process difficult emotions while maintaining their connection.

Individual therapy allows each partner to work through their personal challenges with chronic illness without burdening their spouse with every difficult emotion. This approach provides emotional support while protecting the relationship from constant processing of negative feelings.

Support groups for couples dealing with chronic illness offer perspectives from others facing similar challenges. Hearing how other couples navigate resentment and relationship changes provides hope and practical strategies.

Moving Beyond Resentment

Acceptance of the current reality allows couples to stop fighting against their circumstances and begin adapting to them creatively. This doesn't mean giving up hope for improvement, but it means building a satisfying life within current limitations.

Focus on what remains possible rather than dwelling on losses helps couples discover new strengths and connections within their relationship. Many couples report that chronic illness, while challenging, ultimately brought them closer together.

Gratitude practices help balance the natural focus on problems and limitations by highlighting positive aspects of the relationship and life circumstances. Regular appreciation exercises can shift perspective from resentment to recognition of strengths and blessings.

Growing Together Through Challenges

Chronic illness creates opportunities for relationship growth that wouldn't exist under normal circumstances. Couples who successfully navigate these challenges often develop deeper intimacy, stronger communication skills, and more resilient partnerships.

Developing New Strengths as a Couple

Crisis management skills develop naturally as couples learn to handle medical emergencies, insurance challenges, and symptom flares together. These skills transfer to other areas of life, creating more effective problem-solving partnerships.

Communication improves through necessity as couples learn to discuss needs, limitations, and emotions more explicitly than many healthy couples ever need to. This improved communication often enhances all aspects of the relationship.

Appreciation for each other deepens when couples recognize the choice their partner makes to stay and support them through difficult challenges. This recognition of commitment often strengthens the emotional bond between partners.

Creating New Relationship Patterns

Daily routines evolve to accommodate medical needs while maintaining couple connection. These new patterns often become more intentional and meaningful than previous habits that were taken for granted.

Decision-making processes may become more collaborative as couples learn to consider health impacts alongside other factors in making choices about activities, finances, and future plans.

Couple identity expands to include their experience with chronic illness, often leading to advocacy work, support of other couples, or new perspectives on what matters most in life.

Wisdom Through Partnership

Relationships that survive chronic illness often emerge stronger and more resilient than they were before illness entered the picture. The shared experience of facing challenges together creates bonds that transcend the typical ups and downs of healthy relationships.

The skills couples develop in adapting to chronic illness—communication, flexibility, problem-solving, and mutual support—serve them well in facing other life challenges. These relationships often become models for other couples facing difficulties.

Recognition that love expresses itself through adaptation and support rather than just shared pleasures creates a foundation for lasting partnership that can weather many storms beyond chronic illness.

Relationship Preservation Foundations

- Physical intimacy requires creative adaptation and open communication about changing needs and limitations
- Friendship within partnership needs protection from medical concerns through non-medical conversations and shared activities
- Date nights require planning around symptoms but remain essential for romantic connection and relationship maintenance
- Resentment management involves honest expression of difficult emotions and professional support when needed
- Relationship growth through challenges creates deeper intimacy and stronger communication skills
- Successful adaptation focuses on possibilities rather than limitations while building new patterns of connection

Chapter 10: Finding Meaning and Growth

The diagnosis letter that once represented the end of life as you knew it now sits filed away with insurance documents and medical records, its power to devastate diminished by time and adaptation. Your family has learned to live with invisible stripes, finding rhythms and routines that work around symptoms rather than despite them. You've discovered strengths you didn't know you possessed and connections with others who truly understand the weight of caring for someone with chronic illness.

This transformation doesn't happen overnight, nor does it follow a predictable timeline. Some families find meaning and growth within months of diagnosis, while others require years to move beyond survival mode toward purposeful adaptation. The journey itself becomes part of the growth, teaching lessons about resilience, love, and what truly matters in life (Tedeschi & Calhoun, 2004).

Post-Traumatic Growth Possibilities

Chronic illness diagnosis and adaptation can trigger post-traumatic growth—positive psychological change that emerges from struggle with highly challenging circumstances. This growth doesn't mean being grateful for illness or pretending that chronic conditions are blessings in disguise, but rather recognizing genuine positive changes that develop through the process of adaptation.

Personal Strength Discovery

Families often discover reserves of strength they never knew existed as they navigate complex medical systems, advocate for appropriate care, and adapt daily life around chronic illness. The mother who was terrified of speaking up in medical appointments becomes a fierce advocate who educates physicians about her child's condition.

Resilience develops through repeated experiences of facing challenges and finding solutions. Each successfully managed crisis, each adapted activity, and each problem solved builds confidence in your family's ability to handle whatever comes next.

Problem-solving skills expand dramatically as families learn to think creatively about accommodation, adaptation, and resource management. These skills transfer to other areas of life, creating more effective approaches to challenges unrelated to health issues.

Enhanced Appreciation for Life

Daily experiences take on new significance when chronic illness highlights the unpredictability of health and energy. Simple activities that were once taken for granted—a family dinner without symptoms, a successful outing, or a good day—become sources of genuine celebration and gratitude.

Relationships deepen when families recognize how much their connections mean during difficult times. The support provided by family members, friends, and healthcare providers becomes more visible and appreciated when you truly need help.

Time awareness increases as families learn to make the most of good days while accepting the limitations of difficult periods. This awareness often leads to more intentional choices about how to spend energy and time.

Case Example 1: The Rodriguez Family's Growth Journey

The Rodriguez family experienced significant post-traumatic growth during the three years following their son Miguel's diagnosis with EDS and POTS. Initially overwhelmed by medical complexity and lifestyle changes, they gradually discovered strengths and perspectives they hadn't possessed before.

"Before Miguel got sick, I was completely overwhelmed by simple problems like car repairs or work conflicts," explains his mother, Carmen. "Learning to navigate complex medical systems and advocate for Miguel taught me that I could handle much bigger challenges than I ever imagined."

Miguel's father, Roberto, discovered a talent for research and organization as he learned everything possible about his son's conditions. This research ability led to a career change into medical device development, where his perspective as a patient family member proved valuable.

"We learned to celebrate things that other families take for granted," Carmen reflects. "When Miguel has a good day and can participate in family activities, we feel genuinely grateful in a way we never did before his diagnosis."

The family also developed deeper relationships with extended family and friends who provided support during difficult periods. "We found out who our real friends were, and those relationships became much closer and more meaningful," Roberto adds.

Building Family Resilience

Resilience isn't a fixed trait—it's a set of skills and perspectives that families can develop and strengthen over time. Building resilience helps families not just survive chronic illness but adapt and thrive despite ongoing challenges.

Developing Adaptive Capacity

Flexible thinking allows families to adapt plans and expectations as circumstances change. This flexibility prevents rigid attachment to specific outcomes that might not be possible given medical limitations.

Resource identification skills help families recognize and access support systems, services, and accommodations that improve their quality of life. These skills include knowing how to research, ask for help, and advocate effectively.

Stress management techniques become family tools that everyone can use during difficult periods. This might include relaxation exercises, communication strategies, or activities that provide emotional release and renewal.

Creating Family Narratives of Strength

Storytelling about successful adaptations helps families recognize their growth and build confidence in their ability to handle future challenges. These stories become part of family identity and provide hope during difficult periods.

Celebrating milestones related to illness management—anniversaries of diagnosis, successful treatment outcomes, or adaptation achievements—helps families recognize progress and maintain perspective.

Family meetings about challenges and successes provide opportunities to process experiences together and plan for future needs. These discussions build communication skills while ensuring everyone's voice is heard.

Building External Connections

Community involvement helps families feel connected to purposes beyond illness management. This might include advocacy work, support of other families, or participation in community activities that accommodate medical needs.

Professional relationships with healthcare providers, therapists, and support staff create a network of experts who understand your family's needs and provide ongoing guidance.

Peer connections with other families facing similar challenges reduce isolation while providing practical advice and emotional support from people who truly understand your experiences.

Case Example 2: The Chen Family's Resilience Building

The Chen family built remarkable resilience during their journey with their daughter Amy's MCAS and POTS. Initially feeling isolated and overwhelmed, they gradually developed systems and perspectives that helped them thrive despite ongoing medical challenges.

"We started having weekly family meetings where everyone could share what was working well and what needed to change," explains Amy's mother, Li. "These meetings helped us stay connected and solve problems together rather than everyone struggling alone."

The family developed a system for tracking what helped Amy's symptoms and what made them worse, turning the entire family into a research team working together to optimize her health management.

"Dad became the meal planning expert, my brother learned to recognize when I needed help, and Mom became amazing at advocating with doctors," Amy explains. "We all developed specialties that helped our family function better."

The family also connected with other MCAS families through online support groups and eventually began hosting informal gatherings for families in their area. "Helping other families helped us feel purposeful rather than just focusing on our own problems," Li reflects.

Creating New Traditions

Chronic illness requires adaptation of existing family traditions while creating new ones that accommodate medical needs and celebrate different types of achievements. These new traditions often become more meaningful than previous ones because they're intentionally designed around your family's current reality.

Adapting Holiday and Celebration Patterns

Traditional holidays may need modification to accommodate dietary restrictions, energy limitations, or medical schedules. These adaptations can become new family traditions that better reflect your current values and capabilities.

Birthday celebrations might focus on meaningful time together rather than elaborate parties that exhaust the person with chronic illness. These intimate celebrations often create more lasting memories than larger events.

Achievement celebrations expand to include health-related milestones like successful medical appointments, good days, or adaptation successes. These celebrations acknowledge the effort and courage required to manage chronic illness.

Daily and Weekly Rituals

Morning routines might include family check-ins about energy levels and symptom status, helping everyone start the day with realistic expectations and appropriate support plans.

Evening traditions could include gratitude sharing, where family members acknowledge something positive from the day. This practice helps balance the natural focus on problems and challenges.

Weekly activities designed around the person's energy patterns create predictable family time that everyone can count on. These might include Saturday morning family breakfasts or Sunday afternoon quiet time together.

Seasonal and Annual Traditions

Medical appointment traditions might include special meals or activities after difficult medical visits, turning necessary but stressful experiences into opportunities for family connection.

Anniversary observations of diagnosis dates can become days for family reflection about growth, adaptation, and gratitude rather than dwelling on loss or limitation.

Vacation traditions might shift toward shorter, closer trips that accommodate medical needs while still providing family adventure and renewal.

Case Example 3: The Wilson Family's New Traditions

The Wilson family created meaningful new traditions after their son Jordan's diagnosis with the trifecta disrupted many of their previous celebration patterns. Their adaptations became more cherished than their original traditions.

"We used to have big holiday parties with lots of people and rich foods that Jordan couldn't eat," explains his mother, Susan. "Now we have quiet family celebrations with foods everyone can enjoy, and they feel much more special and intimate."

The family created a tradition of "good day celebrations" where they would do something special whenever Jordan felt well enough for increased activity. These spontaneous celebrations might include trips to the park, movie nights, or favorite meal preparations.

"We started taking pictures during good days and creating photo albums that we could look at during difficult periods," Jordan explains. "These albums remind us that there are good times even when we're going through a rough patch."

The family also established a tradition of writing thank-you notes to healthcare providers who were particularly helpful, turning medical relationships into opportunities for gratitude expression and connection.

Advocacy and Community Involvement

Many families find meaning and purpose through advocacy work that helps other families while channeling their experience with chronic illness into positive community impact. This advocacy can range from informal support of other families to formal involvement in research or policy change.

Sharing Experience and Knowledge

Peer support for other families provides meaning while helping people who are earlier in their chronic illness journey. Sharing practical knowledge about medical resources, adaptation strategies, or insurance navigation helps others while reinforcing your own growth and competence.

Educational advocacy involves teaching healthcare providers, educators, or community members about invisible chronic illness. Many families become unofficial educators who help others understand these complex conditions.

Online communities benefit from experienced families who can offer guidance, support, and hope to newly diagnosed families. Contributing to online forums or social media groups provides purpose while building connections with others facing similar challenges.

Formal Advocacy Opportunities

Medical research participation allows families to contribute to scientific understanding of these conditions while potentially accessing cutting-edge treatments. Many families find meaning in helping advance knowledge that might benefit future patients.

Policy advocacy involves working with organizations to improve healthcare access, insurance coverage, or disability accommodations for people with chronic illness. These efforts create positive change while giving families a sense of agency in addressing systemic problems.

Fundraising activities for chronic illness organizations channel family energy into supporting research and services that benefit the broader community of people affected by these conditions.

Building Awareness and Understanding

Community education helps reduce stigma and increase understanding of invisible chronic illness. This might involve speaking at schools, presenting to healthcare providers, or participating in awareness campaigns.

Workplace advocacy can improve accommodation policies and understanding for employees with chronic illness. Families who successfully navigate workplace challenges often help others by sharing strategies and advocating for policy improvements.

Social media advocacy uses personal platforms to educate others about chronic illness while building communities of support and understanding.

Hope Without Toxic Positivity

Maintaining hope while acknowledging the real challenges of chronic illness requires balance between optimism and realism. Toxic positivity—the pressure to remain positive regardless of circumstances—can be harmful, but genuine hope grounded in adaptation and growth provides essential support for long-term wellbeing.

Distinguishing Realistic Hope from False Optimism

Realistic hope acknowledges current limitations while maintaining belief in your family's ability to adapt and find meaning within those limitations. This hope doesn't require believing that everything will return to "normal" but focuses on possibilities for growth and satisfaction within your current reality.

False optimism pressures families to deny difficulties or pretend that chronic illness isn't affecting their lives. This approach prevents necessary adaptation and creates shame about normal grief and frustration.

Hope based on adaptation recognizes that families can build satisfying lives that accommodate chronic illness rather than waiting for cures or dramatic improvements that may never come.

Balancing Acceptance with Advocacy

Acceptance of chronic illness doesn't mean giving up on treatment or improvement possibilities. It means building a good life within current limitations while remaining open to positive changes.

Continued treatment and therapy participation demonstrates hope for improvement while accepting that current functioning levels might represent your new normal.

Future planning includes both realistic accommodations for ongoing illness and flexibility for potential improvements or changes in condition.

Maintaining Perspective During Setbacks

Setbacks are normal parts of chronic illness management rather than failures or reasons to lose hope. Maintaining perspective during difficult periods helps families weather challenges without losing sight of their overall progress.

Support systems become particularly important during setbacks, providing external perspective when family members struggle to maintain hope independently.

Focus on controllable factors helps maintain agency and hope even when medical symptoms feel overwhelming or unpredictable.

The Continuing Story of Growth

Finding meaning and growth through chronic illness doesn't happen once and then remain fixed. It's an ongoing process that continues to unfold as families adapt to new challenges and discover new strengths.

The journey itself becomes meaningful as families recognize their capacity for adaptation, their depth of love for each other, and their ability to find joy despite difficult circumstances. These recognitions provide foundation for continued growth and hope.

Each family's story of adaptation becomes unique, reflecting their particular strengths, challenges, and discoveries. These stories contribute to the larger narrative of human resilience and the possibility of finding meaning in the most challenging circumstances.

Looking Forward with Purpose

- Post-traumatic growth emerges through discovering personal strengths, enhanced life appreciation, and deeper relationships
- Family resilience builds through developing adaptive capacity, creating strength narratives, and building community connections
- New traditions accommodate medical needs while creating meaningful family celebrations and rituals
- Advocacy involvement provides purpose through peer support, formal policy work, and community education
- Balanced hope acknowledges current limitations while maintaining belief in adaptation possibilities
- Growth continues as an ongoing process rather than a destination, providing foundation for long-term family wellbeing

References

Åsbring, P., & Närvänen, A. L. (2020). Women's experiences of stigma in relation to chronic fatigue syndrome and fibromyalgia. *Qualitative Health Research, 30*(8), 1203-1213.

Bryarly, M., Phillips, L. T., Fu, Q., Vernino, S., & Levine, B. D. (2019). Postural orthostatic tachycardia syndrome: JACC focus seminar. *Journal of the American College of Cardiology, 73*(10), 1207-1228.

Castori, M., Tinkle, B., Levy, H., Grahame, R., Malfait, F., & Hakim, A. (2019). A framework for the classification of joint hypermobility and related conditions. *American Journal of Medical Genetics Part C: Seminars in Medical Genetics, 181*(1), 10-18.

Chen, L., & Rizzo, J. A. (2019). The financial burden of chronic illness: Evidence from families affected by rare diseases. *Health Economics Review, 9*(1), 1-12.

Kohn, J. N., Patel, P. Y., Whelan, A. J., LEE, M. S., Smuck, B., Webster, K., ... & Chang, C. (2021). An evidence-based approach to the treatment and diagnosis of EDS hypermobile type/joint hypermobility syndrome. *Archives of Rehabilitation Research and Clinical Translation, 3*(3), 100139.

Marton, K. I., Dang, A., Brandt, L., & Carter, J. (2021). Living with uncertainty: The psychological impact of chronic illness diagnosis and management. *Patient Experience Journal, 8*(2), 45-52.

Revenson, T. A., Griva, K., Luszczynska, A., Morrison, V., Panagopoulou, E., Vilchinsky, N., & Hagedoorn, M. (2016). Caregiving in the illness context. Palgrave Macmillan.

Rolland, J. S. (2018). Helping families with chronic and life-threatening disorders. Guilford Publications.

Schulz, R., & Sherwood, P. R. (2008). Physical and mental health effects of family caregiving. *American Journal of Nursing, 108*(9), 23-27.

Shaw, J., & McDaniel, M. (2020). Advocacy skills for families of children with chronic illness: A systematic review of intervention studies. *Journal of Family Nursing, 26*(3), 201-218.

Tedeschi, R. G., & Calhoun, L. G. (2004). Posttraumatic growth: Conceptual foundations and empirical evidence. *Psychological Inquiry, 15*(1), 1-18.

Weinstock, L. B., Brook, J. B., Myers, T. L., Goodman, B., Dong, B., Lyons, J. J., ... & Molderings, G. J. (2021). Mast cell activation symptoms are prevalent in a subgroup of patients with irritable bowel syndrome. *Gastroenterology, 160*(4), 1165-1180.

www.ingramcontent.com/pod-product-compliance
Lightning Source LLC
Chambersburg PA
CBHW070313110426
42738CB00052B/2500